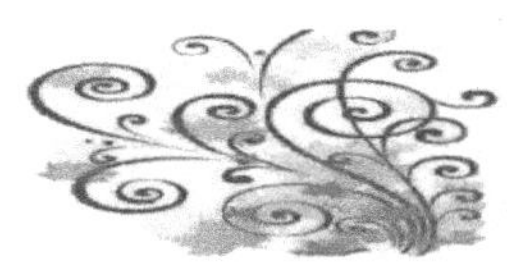

EATING GUIDE: EASIEST WAY TO BURN FAT AND LOSE WEIGHT IN 28 DAYS, STAY HEALTHY, AND LIVE LONGER

by

JANET SMITH

Dedicated to all lovers of my humble works

Foreword

I've always known Janet Smith to be shy and introspective. Big mistake. With her first ever nutrition book: 'Poached Eggs: These Little Tips Mean A Lot' and then this one, I've changed the way I see her. She is an authority in Nutrition. An exceptional cook, whom I bet, has a thousand and one food recipes stuck in her head.

This little book gives insight to all you need just to stay healthy and in shape. Therein are topics that mean a lot to us like ketogenic diets (with complete recipes on how to prepare five great ketogenic meals in an easy to understand manner. And the benefits, the myths, the limit, and side effects of ketogenic diets), weight loss regimen and meal plan, weight loss food recipes, and matters relating to egg poaching.

This book is indeed a life saver.

Edwin Harris

(Freelancer and Health and Nutrition specialist)

TABLE OF CONTENTS

Introduction

Section 1

THE COMPLETE KETOGENIC DIET FOR STARTERS: ESSENTIAL GUIDE TO KETO LIFESTYLE

Section 2

28 DAYS WEIGHT LOSS PLAN: DON'T STARVE. DON'T SUFFER COUNTING CALORIES. EAT THESE NEW FAST METABOLISM DIETS

Introduction

Chapter One

Difficulty of weight loss regimens

How will I feel when I begin this diet plan?

How many calories should I eat?

What if I feel hungry?

What if I miss a meal on the plan?

Shopping List for the one month Diet Plan

Chapter Two

Diet plan (from day 1–28)

Chapter Three

Physical exercises that will hasten up body metabolism

Chapter Four

19 Best Recipes for 28 days Weight Loss Plan (each listed and explained for easy execution)

Section 3

NINETEEN BEST KETOGENIC RECIPES OF ALL TIMES

Diets that will really help you lose weight

Section 4

REBRAND YOUR LIFE: DRINKS THAT WILL BOOST METABOLISM IN 28 DAYS

Chapter One

- **Pear juice**

Benefits of pear juice

How to make pear juice

How to store pear juice

Chapter Two

- **Coffee**

Reasons you should start taking coffee

Chapter Three

- **Green Coffee**

Benefits of taking Green coffee

Quantity of Green coffee to take

Methods of preparing Green coffee

Ingredients for making Green coffee

Facts to keep in mind about Green coffee

Section 5

POACHED EGGS: THESE LITTLE SECRETS MEAN A LOT

Chapter One

Eggs and the Methods of Cooking

Chapter Two

Poached Eggs and Your Health

Chapter Three

Tools for Poaching Eggs

Chapter Four: How to Make Garlic bread with Poached Eggs

Chapter Five: Pasta with Poached Eggs

Chapter Six: Poached Eggs and Bacon Salad

Chapter Seven: Making Money with Poached Eggs

Section 1

THE COMPLETE KETOGENIC DIET FOR STARTERS: ESSENTIAL GUIDE TO KETO LIFESTYLE

Introduction

In a time like this, when junk foods are available at every corner, when we feel more disposed to make quick-fix foods, it becomes quite important to talk about our diet and how it affects our overall being. In this section of the book, we will focus on ketogenic diet; the benefits, myths, and recipes. You'll be getting some really good advice on what to eat on a keto diet.

Your weight loss dream is not farfetched. The selected recipes have been researched and will work wonders. Please read.

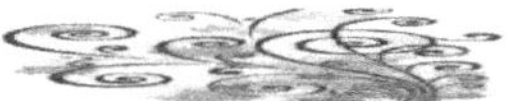

Chapter One

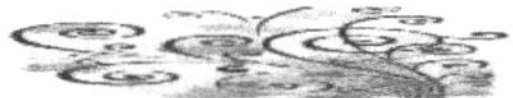

WHAT IS A KETOGENIC DIET?

My mother, at one point, was overweight. She used to love eggs. I wasn't sure the eggs made her to blow up anyway. But I was sure she didn't like those extra chunks of flesh and weight. The supplements.. The regimens.. The diet plans. She was exhausted when none worked. While I was reading a nutrition book, I came across a section on ketogenic diet recipes. I said to myself, 'Janet, You've got to try these out on mom.'

The quirky thing is that she became skeptical of everything anyone suggested including when I suggested some ketogenic diets. She was stubborn.

And I told her she didn't have to pay for my services. She laughed and eventually became willing to try out something from her only daughter. In late 2016, we began a keto meal plan. By February 2017, my mother looked in the mirror and said: 'Jane, I'm twelve years younger.'

Wait a minute, what's a ketogenic diet?

A ketogenic diet is also known as low carbohydrate diet or low carbohydrate-high fat diet. This diet helps the body to produce ketones in the liver which the body eventually converts into energy. It is only normal that when you eat something high in carbohydrates, it spurs your body to produce insulin and glucose.

Glucose- this is just the easiest molecule that your body can convert and use as energy.

Insulin– this is produced to help process the glucose in your bloodstream. It does that by circulating glucose around the body.

Now, since we have seen that glucose is being used as a primary source of energy, the fats in the body are not needed. Therefore, they are stored. In fact even when your intake of carbohydrate is high, the body will still use glucose as the main form of energy. So should you lower your intake of carbohydrates? Well, the moment you lower carbohydrate intake, the body is induced into a state called Ketosis.

What is Ketosis?

This is a natural process initiated by the body to keep us alive when food intake is very low. During this state the body produces ketones by breaking down fats in the liver. The essence of a well maintained keto diet is to drag your body into this metabolic state of fats breakdown. Some may consider starvation of fatty foods as an option because they want the body to produce ketones so they can take down more fats. That wouldn't help achieve what you want. It is rather starvation of carbohydrates that will.

Ordinarily, the body is incredibly adaptive to what you force into it- if you overfeed it with fats and reduce carbohydrates it will begin to burn ketones as a primary source of energy.

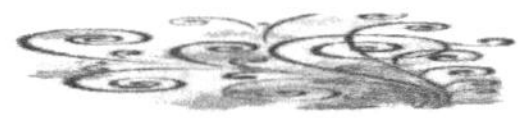

Chapter Two

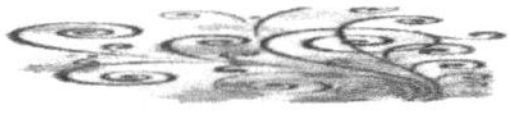

BENEFITS OF A KETOGENIC DIET

I actually tried some of the keto recipes that I found in the nutrition book I was reading, on my mother. I can bet that she eventually was healthier, smarter, and above all, she lost quite some pounds of flesh. I'm heck serious. I couldn't believe it. I had been working with faith. Now, what I realized was that keto diets were perfect for weight loss but whether it will work on you or not depends on the mind.

The benefits of ketogenic diets are quite numerous. We are going to be taking a close look at each of them.

1. Mental Focus

The stress of life often leads us astray when it comes to what we eat. We just are too tired to take a second thought at what goes into our bodies. As a result, we may face decline in energy levels at work. In fact one of the reasons why one finds it difficult to concentrate on a task is an improper diet. Ketones are a great source of fuel for the brain. By lowering you carbohydrate intake, you avoid a whole lot of big spikes in your blood sugar. This can help you focus and concentrate better. There is a reduction in the excess neurons in the brain thus leading to mental focus. To help your day, you could start every day with a cup of ketoproof coffee (I personally enjoy this every morning).

2. Weight Loss

I decided to make this come second but I bet, for many, it is the first reason they are trying a ketogenic diet. The fats in the body are essentially used by the ketogenic diet as a good source of energy. Your insulin levels drop greatly thereby turning your body into a fat burning machine. In other words, storage of excess fat is denied in the body. It is only wise to conclude that keto diets eventually lead to weight loss.

3. Blood Sugar Control

Blood sugar levels are naturally lowered by ketones due to the type of foods that goes into your system. Studies have shown that ketogenic diets can effectively help to manage and prevent diabetes better than low-calorie diets. Diabetes patients should make it a priority to incorporate ketogenic diets in their food roster.

4. Acne

Do you have acne? Or does your skin look unattractive? There are a whole lot factors that can cause skin irritations but for many, Ketogenic diets are a key solution. One study shows how lesions and skin inflammations dropped when people with them switched to ketogenic diets. Another study shows that there may be a connection between a high consumption of carbohydrates and acne. However if you have acne, in addition to keto diet, it would be beneficial to reduce intake of dairy products and strictly follow a skin cleaning regimen.

5. Insulin Resistance

Type II diabetes can result from insulin resistance if not managed with care. Several researches have shown that ketogenic diets can help lower insulin levels to a healthy range. Even those who are athletic can benefit immensely from insulin optimization on ketogenic diets especially by eating foods high in omega-3 fatty acids.

6. Epilepsy

Since the early 1900's, ketogenic diets have been used to treat patients with epilepsy. It has recorded huge success both then and now. Today, it is one of the most widely used therapies for children who have uncontrolled epilepsy. The good thing about this diet is that it allows an epileptic patient to still take few medications while offering excellent hold on the patient.

7. Increased Energy

This point cannot be overemphasized. Keto diets are a reliable source of energy.

8. Full

Ketogenic diets can keep your stomach full for longer hours. The fatty contents are generally satisfying and can keep you less hungry while providing your body with energy.

Are you beginning to consider including ketogenic diets in your food roster? That'd be great, absolutely great. But then what should you eat on a ketogenic diet. The next chapter will discuss this.

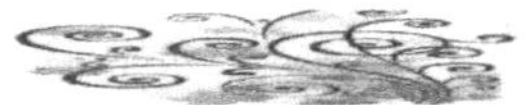

Chapter Three

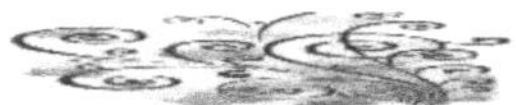

WHAT TO EAT ON A KETOGENIC DIET

Beginning a keto diet is quite easy. But you will need to plan ahead. You should include it on your food roster, if you have one. What you eat largely depends on how quick you want to get into a ketogenic state. The truth is, the more restrictive you are on your carbohydrates, the faster you will achieve the desire buried in your heart.

You would want to ensure that your carbohydrate consumption is limited. It should be coming mostly from nuts, diaries, and vegetables. Greatly avoid carbohydrates that are refined such as wheat (pasta, bread, cereals), starch (beans, legumes, potatoes), or fruits. Some of the fruits you may wish to eat include star fruit, avocado, and berries.

What you should not eat

It is vital that you strictly keep off from the following:

Sugar – marple syrup, agave, etc.

Tubers – yams, potatoes, etc.

Grains – corn, rice, wheat, cereal, etc.

Fruits – oranges, apples, bananas, etc.

What you should eat

Try to incorporate the following in your diet:

High Fat Diary – high fat cream, butter, hard cheese, etc.

Meat – fish, poultry, eggs, beef, lab, etc.

Avocados and berries – blackberries, raspberries, and other berries that have low glyceric impact on the body

Nuts and Seeds – sunflower seeds, walnuts, macadamias, etc.

Leafy Greens – kale, spinach, etc.

Sweeteners – saturated fats, coconut oil, high fat salad dressing, etc.

Important

Keep in mind that keto is high in fat, moderate in protein, and on the low side in carbohydrate. So doing a little math, your nutrients intake should be around

Fats: 70%

Protein: 25%

Carbohydrate: 5%

Normally, anywhere between 25- 30g of net carbohydrate is recommended for everyday dieting. The lower you keep your carbohydrate intake and glucose levels, the better the overall results. If the reason you are on keto diet is to lose weight, it will be worthwhile to keep track of your total carbohydrate and net carbohydrate.

Net carbohydrates are your total dietary carbohydrate minus the total fiber. For example you want to eat I cup of brocilli, there are a total of 6g of carbohydrates in 1 cup, and 2g of fiber in the same 1 cup. So we have a total of 6g carbohydrate and 2g dietary fiber.

To get our net carbohydrate, you will have to minus the 2kg dietary fiber from the 6kg carbohydrate. This will give you 4kg net carbohydrate.

If you oftentimes find yourself hungry during the day, you could snack on something like seeds, nuts, cheeses, or peanut butter to manage your appetite. (Snacking regularly can delay weight loss in the long term).

Vegetables on a Ketogenic Diet

Leafy and dark green is just the right choice for vegetables. Most of what you eat should be protein with vegetables, and an extra side of fat.

You can also consider Chicken breast in olive oil, with broccoli and cheese. And steak topped with a knob of butter and a part of spinach sautéed in olive oil.

In the chapters that follow, I'd list out one-by-one the keto recipes that worked on my mother. I bet you, they are really effective and can help you trim down quicker than you had expected.

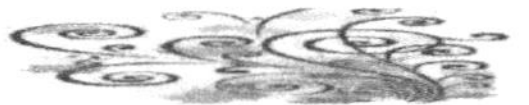

Chapter Four

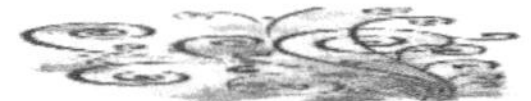

KETO TUNA CASSEROLE

This is one of my favourite comfort dinners during the cold. My mother knew how to make it well. It was quite easy. I learnt how to make it before I turned fourteen. Funny enough, we weren't eating it often. At the time, mom and I had no idea this meal could help in weight loss. I only discovered this hidden benefit six years later after completing a course on Nutrition. Tuna Casserole is made usually, with some carbohydrate vegetables like peas. I decided to swap those out for this recipe for some keto- friendly vegetables like mushrooms and a little amount of carrots. Then I use shirataki noodles in lieu of pasta noodles. But if you can't reach shirataki noodles, zucchini noodles are a great alternative.

The good thing about the recipe, is that it is incredibly easy to prepare, with just a little of your time to spend.

What you will need:

½ Cup chopped carrots

2 tablespoons butter

½ cup chopped green onions

½ cup chopped mushrooms

4 packages (226kg each) shirataki noodles

½ teaspoon xanthan gum

2 cups heavy whipping cream

½ cup shredded cheddar cheese

2 cans (146kg each) tuna

Salt and pepper

How to cook

- Melt you butter in a deep pot over medium heat
- Add to the green onions, carrots and mushrooms
- Sauté the vegetables for 3–5 minutes
- Sprinkle the xanthan gum over the vegetables
- Add your cream quickly and stir. Ensure to keep on the heat until you begin to see bubbles.

- Place your shirataki noodles in a casserole dish and stir the cream mixture into the noodles

- Mix in your flaked tuna and cheddar cheese

- Bake at 350 degrees Fahrenheit for about 35 minutes.

Your keto Tuna Casserole is ready.

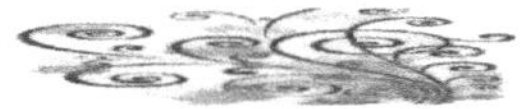

Chapter Five

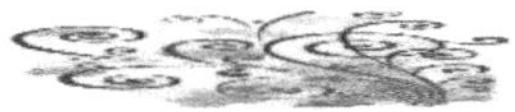

CHRISTMAS WREATH MERINGUE

This is a great holiday dessert that you and your family will really enjoy. It is fashioned to look like a Pavlova. Since there is no sugar, the meringue does not crisp up. Instead, this meringue dessert holds its shape very firm to the touch yet it is almost like marshmallow in texture and taste. The cream and fruits added, makes it festive.

What you will need

100g strawberries

100g raspberries

300g heavy whipping cream

100g blueberries

½ tablespoon powdered erythritol

50g allulose

½ teaspoon white vinegar

1 teaspoon vanilla bean paste

Sprigs of mint or rosemary (this will help garnish).

How to Cook

- Prepare the fruits and keep aside
- Preheat oven to 225 degrees Fahrenheit.
- Prepare meringue ingredients
- Put the egg whites in a bowl and whisk until soft peaks

- Add allulose, little by little, until stiff and glossy
- Stir in vinegar
- Make a shallow trench in the meringue. This will serve as a well for the cream and fruits to sit in.
- Bake for 30 minutes. When due, turn off the oven but leave the meringue inside to cool and dry.
- Add allulose and cream to a bowl and whip until it become s fluffy after which you can add the vanilla bean paste.
- Whip and refrigerate the paste until ready to use
- Finally, spoon chilled cream on the trench. Then arrange fruits and decorate them with the mint leaves or rosemary. Dust with powdered erythritol.
- Cut into desired wedges and serve.

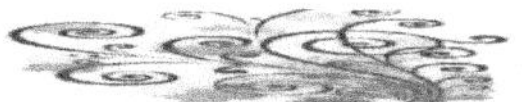

Chapter Six

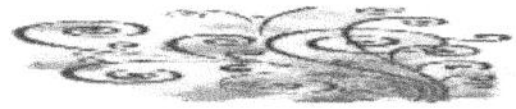

SAUSAGE ZUCCHINI BOATS

This is quite easy. Not just easy but delicious as well. The smells are stuffed with sausage. You can add meat, any kind you prefer, as long as it is ground beef, lamb, chicken, or any other choice you make. The recipe is perfect. Kids will love this, trust me. This must be a plus to the keto value.

What you will need:

1 pound ground sausage

1 cup shredded cheddar cheese

1 tablespoon minced garlic

½ cup chicken

¾ cup chicken broth

¾ medium onion, chopped

2 medium zucchini

Salt and pepper

1 teaspoon paprika

½ teaspoon red pepper flakes

1 teaspoon dried oregano

How to cook:

- Cut your zucchini in two
- Scoop out the zucchini with a spoon or melon-baller so it becomes like a shell for the fillings

- It is time to chop up the zucchini that you scooped out of the skins.

- Sauté your onions, garlic, and scooped zucchini over medium heat

- Add your spices and the sausage

- Once the sausage is cooked, add in your cheese and keep cooking until it melts.

- Cut the cooked zucchini and sausage mixture in two among the zucchini shells

- Add some more cheese and place into a casserole dish

- Put in your chicken broth into the bottom of the dish.

- Allow to bake for 30 minutes at 350 degrees Fahrenheit.

Your Zucchini Boats are ready to be consumed.

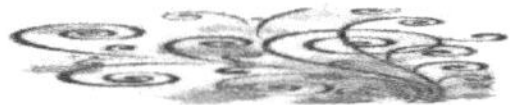

Chapter Seven

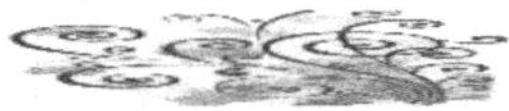

VEGETARIAN THREE CHEESE QUICHE STUFFED PEPPERS

A few things may stroll into your mind when you think of making a quiche. You may begin to feel oh no, it is time consuming, complicated, and so on. It may not be your idea of an easy keto diet. Well, this recipe I'm about to give you is absolutely easy. I mean it; very easy. The good thing about this diet is that it is vegetarian friendly and satisfying. This is one of my choicest dinners. The taste of lightly seasoned egg that is made fluffy, mixed with full fat ricotta, mozzarella, and the bite of shredded Parmesan are just mind blowing. Not to even mention the leaves of fresh spinach which vegetarians will love for the light green boost.

What you will need:

4 large eggs

2 tablespoon Parmesan cheese

2 medium bell peppers, cut in half and seeds taken out

½ cup ricotta cheese

½ cup grated Parmesan cheese

1 teaspoon garlic powder

¼ cup baby spinach leaves

¼ teaspoon dried parsley

½ cup shredded mozzarella

How to cook

- Prepare the peppers by cutting them into four. Ensure that you take out the seeds
- Heat oven to 375 degrees Fahrenheit
- Blend the three cheese, eggs, parsley, and garlic powder in a small food processor
- Pour the egg mixture into each pepper, until it gets just below the rim. Place some baby spinach leaves on top and stir with a fork, pushing them under the egg.
- Cover and leave to bake for about 40 minutes or until the egg is set.
- Sprinkle with Parmesan cheese and broil for 4 minutes or until the tops turn brown.

This recipe makes a total of four single servings. Each of the serving comes out with:

Protein- 17.84g

Calories- 245.5g

Fat- 16.2g

Net carbohydrate- 5.97

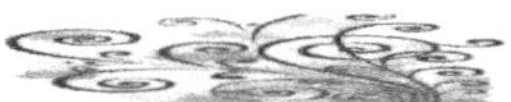

Chapter Eight

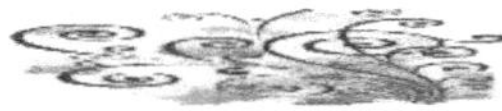

CHICKEN TENDER LAZONE

Is there a chicken dinner you want prepared in a flash, it is Chicken tender Lazone. It is absolutely flavorful. This meal involves pan searing smoky chicken tenders in butter to be served with noodles. It is a perfect keto diet if you want something really quick for dinner. This is tasty. Do not be surprised if you catch someone trying to scrap out the last bits of sauce out of the pan and stuffing in the mouth.

What you will need:

1 cup heavy whipping cream

¼ teaspoon xanthan gum

2 teaspoon smoked paprika

¾ teaspoon garlic powder

½ teaspoon onion powder

½ teaspoon dried basil

½ teaspoon dried oregano

I tablespoon olive oil

Salt and pepper

5 tablespoon unsalted butter

1.25 pounds (8 pieces) chicken tenderloins

1.25 pounds spiral zucchini

How to cook:

- Combine the smoked paparika, garlic powder p, cayenne pepper, onion powder, dried oregano, dried basil, and some pepper and salt

- Place your chicken tenderloins in a medium sized bowl and pour the tablespoon of olive oil and seasoning mix. Mix them together

- In a large skillet, melt 3 tablespoon of the butter over medium heat.

- Add the chicken tenderloins and cook for some 3 or 4 minutes. The chicken should get to 165 degrees Fahrenheit. Set them side once they are done.

- Cook the zucchini and season with salt and pepper (to your taste) in the microwave or sauté in another pan. Ensure that excess water is dried.

- Add 2 tablespoon of butter in the skillet you cooked the chicken. Then whisk in the cup of cream.

- Whisk in the xanthan gum also so that the sauce can thicken up.

Serve with the zucchini tossing with noodles while the chicken is on top.

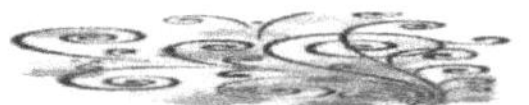

Chapter Nine

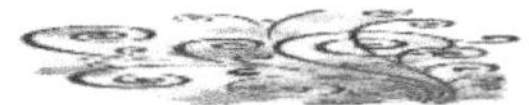

REACHING KETOSIS

Reaching ketosis is not a difficult, painful process. It is quite easy. But at first, it can look confusing especially with all the information out there. I've assured you that the five keto recipes just discussed helped my own mother trim down. It can help you too. But to be really sure you are doing the right thing, below pinpoints all you need to really do to lose weight.

Cut down on protein

Too much protein can lead to lower levels of ketosis. Normally for weight loss, you should eat between 0.6g and 0.8g protein per pound lean body mass.

Cut down on carbohydrate

Do not just focus on net carbohydrate if you really want to achieve ketosis. Limit both net carbs and total carbs. It will do you good to stay below 20g of net carbohydrate and 35g of total carbohydrate.

Drink plenty of water

This fact cannot be overemphasized. Keeping your body hydrated consistently will help regulate your body function and keep hunger under control. At least, you don't get to eat anyhow

Avoid snacking

You really want to reach ketosis right? Then you've got to cut down on snacking. This will help in manage your insulin spikes during the day and quicken weight loss.

Get Enough Exercise

The value of exercising cannot also be overemphasized. Aside regulating blood sugar level and helping in weight loss, exercising in the morning before you eat can really help you get the most of your ketogenic diet.

Signs of reaching Ketosis

If you want to determine whether you're in ketosis, you can, through urine or blood strips (although there are claims that the urine strips are inaccurate and the blood strips can be expensive). So what should you do? How can you decipher you have reached your 'promise land'?

The following signs are pretty helpful

Reduced hunger and increased energy

You will experience a much lower hunger level and feel energized in your daily duties

Frequent urination

Since keto is a natural diuretic, you may pressed to urinate more. Acetoacetate which is a ketone body is excreted in the urine.

Dry mouth

As a result of frequent urination, your mouth tends to become dry and you have increased thirst. In this case, you will have to keep on drinking plenty of water to replenish the salt, potassium and magnesium in your system.

Bad breath

One ketone body that is excreted through our breath is Acetone. It does not smell fine. In fact the person next could sniff and move away. I don't know how best to describe the smell but the nearest could be compared to an overripe fruit or nail polish remover. But not to worry, there's good news: the smell is only temporary and when it goes, it does not resurface.

My mother's smell lasted just a couple of days. I didn't really bother much.

Types of Keto Diets

1. Clinical Ketogenic Diets

This kind of keto diet is for contest goers and bodybuilders. It is taken once a week to carb up and resupply glycogen to the body.

2. Standard Ketogenic Diets

This is the normal keto diet that is familiar to everyone.

3. Targeted Ketogenic Diets

This is a slight variation of the standard ketogenic diet. In this case you take in a little amount of fast-digesting carbohydrate before a workout.

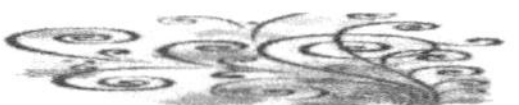

Chapter Ten

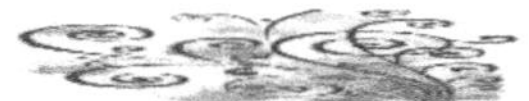

KETOGENIC DIET AND YOUR PHYSICAL PERFORMANCE

It is common to hear people argue that performance is affected when on ketogenic diet. Can that be true? Well in the short run, you may experience little physical performance drops but this will subside over time as you continue to replenish electrolytes, fluids, and adapt to the fat intake.

A study was done on some trained cyclists who were on ketogenic diets for four weeks. From the results, it was clear that their aerobic performance was not compromised at all, and that their muscle mass didn't change, it was just the same as when they began.

However, it is possible to experience performance drops in exercises relating to explosive actions. In that case, you may need to increase your carbohydrate intake a bit. Eating 25-30g of carbohydrate before you train will just do the magic.

Dangers of ketogenic diets

The gospel truth is; there's absolutely nothing that is just perfect and without another side. So what could be the other side of ketogenic diets? The state where ketone production in the body becomes very high is known as **ketoacidosis**. In this case you would need medical intervention. Dangerously high levels of ketone will lead to insulin secretion. However, not to worry, a normal continuous intake of ketogenic diets will not harm you except you have type I diabetes. In this case, insulin level is low.

As a precaution, it will be wise for you to check with your doctor if you intend to start a keto diet. This will help in case you are currently on medications.

If you are starting a ketogenic diet for the first time, you'd most likely experience what we may refer to as **Keto Flu.** You may feel some slight discomfort but that only last a short while.

What are the common side effects on a keto diet?

- Constipation
- Cramps
- Reduced physical performance

- Heart palpitations

What you will never experience on a keto diet (myths)

- Increased Cholesterol
- Gallstones
- Keto Rash
- Hair Loss

In all, my simple suggestion is, keto diets are awesome. Include them in your food roster and enjoy immensely, the taste and health benefits. But if you are taking a medication, please check with your doctor. It is my wish that my readers reach satisfaction and stronger health.

Section 2

28 DAYS WEIGHT LOSS PLAN: DON'T STARVE. DON'T SUFFER COUNTING CALORIES. EAT THESE NEW FAST METABOLISM DIETS

INTRODUCTION

You may have tried many diets or eating plans only to find out how difficult the routine can be with only just a little result to show for it. After all the restrictions, you are still the same; overweight. Though this book targets nutrition that have proved to be effective on weight loss, a few exercise regimens that go a long way in putting our body in shape, burning calories, and foster weight loss, are explained in simple and easy-to-do terms.

Many people, on a regular basis, eat every seemingly good thing they see; junks and other quick-fix foods. And when they eat like this, they oftentimes need supplements and loads of caffeine to keep them throughout the day. Sadly, these quick-fix foods put stress on the body because the body wasn't meant to eat those on a regular basis. The body ends up working too much to ensure that the toxins you have eaten are cleared out. The organ in the body that performs this function is the liver. The liver helps to balance sugar level, break down not –needed hormones, store nutrients, and remove toxins. The moment the liver begins not to work properly because you frequently overload it with toxins from junk foods to clear, problems such as bad skin, tiredness, weight gain, etc., will occur.

Ensure to follow the diet plan in this book for expected results.

CHAPTER ONE

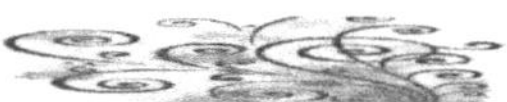

Difficulty with Weight Loss Regimens

I must confess that as a result of your tight schedule and social engagement, strictly following the diets plan in this book may be burdensome. But then you already know what you want; to lose weight. You want this badly, more than anything else. So plan ahead how you can follow this diet plan for optimal results. If you like so much caffeine a day, you may wish to re-adjust to the diet plan I have mapped out. In fact, to be able to give a testimony, you may make serious changes on your eating habits to align to my diet plan. Just as many of those I have helped, including mu mother, I know you will have questions about this diet plan. A few of those probable questions are answered just below. If you have further questions please do not hesitate to contact me via mail or Facebook page. I will be glad to help with your queries.

How will I feel when I begin this diet plan?

For some people, the first seven days will seem to be really tough. You may have to battle with energy loss, dizziness, and headache. So you end up assuming the process is not worth it. Please don't give up. To combat the negative side effects, drink plenty of water every day. At least 2 liters of water will do.

How many calories should I eat?

This plan bothers around wholesome foods that will nourish your body. It does not count calories or low fats; instead you will find yourself eating more foods.

What if I feel hungry?

This guide will help you manage hunger. The diet plan will make you feel less hungry before your next meal. But in a situation where you feel hungry, drink enough water before heading for a light food.

What if I miss a meal on the plan?

While I encourage that you strictly follow this diet plan, I understand stand how circumstances beyond your control may cause you to fall short of the arrangement. Not to worry, get back with the rest of the days. A day or two will not mal the effect of the plan. However, to guarantee quick and expected results stick to the plan religiously.

Shopping List for the one month Diet Plan

The list may seem overwhelming and expensive but it is actually worth the cost. Some people end up spending more money on things that are costly and detrimental to their health. Spending money on health nourishing food should not be a problem.

Meat

Lamb

Pork

Beef

Un-smoked bacon

Gluten free sausages

Eggs

Goose

Chicken

Duck

Seafood

Crab

Cod

Tuna

Pollock

Trout

Mackerel

Shrimp

Salmon

Anchovies

Fruits

Lime

Avocados

Blueberries

Blackberries

Tomatoes

Melon

Peaches

Apples

Lemon

Vegetables

Broccoli

Carrots

Cabbage

Celery

Pecans

Pistachios

Cauliflowers

Brussels sprouts

Asparagus

Fats

Ghee

Grass-fed butter

Avocado oil

Macadamia oil

Extra virgin oil

Nuts

Hazelnuts

Chestnuts

Cashews

Almonds

Brazil nuts

Other things you will need

Almond milk desiccated coconut

Coconut cream (bar)

Coconut milk

Coconut flakes

Grass-fed heavy cream

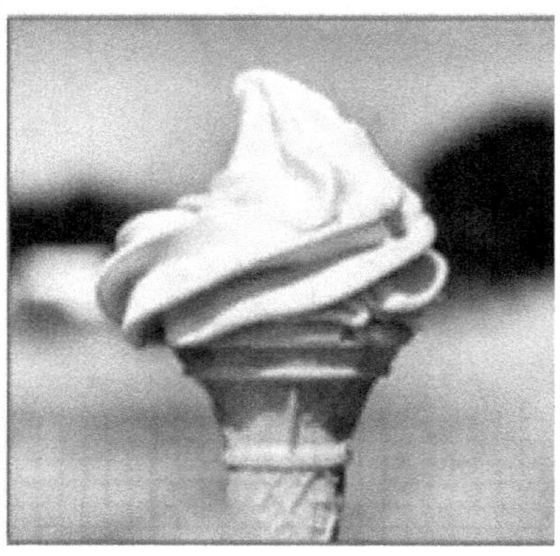

Before you eat this ask yourself: are
the calories actually worth it?

The truth is that becoming overweight or obese is
no longer uncommon, neither is it an uncommon
sight to you to see people who are best-in-shape.
Sincerely speaking, whether it is you or someone
else, being overweight is horrible. You do not look

sexy or attractive in your clothes when you are on the street, or when you are in briefs in the bedroom. My mother was always lacking energy. At fifty-three, she had reached 110kg. It didn't make her happy. I wasn't either. But the good thing is that she's now better. Now weighing 82kg, she definitely has a lot of testimonies.

Enough of the bad look that makes you feel not superior, that makes you feel ashamed of yourself. You must be aware that simple dietary changes can be the solution to your discomfort. Or aren't you? No matter your current weight, there are foods that can help amp up your body's metabolism, causing you to burn more fat and shed some excess pounds. Of course, if you are seeking to make major changes to your body, dietary changes alone are not sufficient you will also need to begin and stick religiously to a regular exercise regimen. But then a good step to start with is to start, with what you eat.

To resolve the issue of what you should eat, consider the following:

Fish is a good source of omega-3 fatty acids and it reduces the amount of leptin in your body. Leptin, plays a key role in your metabolism, by determining whether your body burns calories or stores them as fat. More leptin in your body makes you more likely to store fat, while lower leptin levels makes you more likely to burn fat.

Milk, whole grains and oats can also help burn fat by providing your body with complex carbohydrates and calcium. These complex carbohydrates and calcium help keep your metabolism going by keeping your insulin levels low after you eat. High insulin production can trigger your body to start storing fat; fat in turn, slows metabolism. But if your metabolism keeps moving and the insulin stays low, your body will burn fat more easily. Low-fat yogurt is the best kind of yogurt you should opt for.

Lean beef, turkey, chicken and pork can help you to burn fat. The protein within these lean meats requires more energy to digest. So if you are eating more protein, your body will work harder to digest it, burning more calories and fat. The key, though, is that the meat you eat is lean and relatively void of additives. Cut away any fat or skin that may be on the meat, and minimize–or completely avoid–any marinades or sauces that will pack extra calories into your dish.

Hot peppers, particularly jalapenos, habaneras and cayenne's, work wonders by boosting your heart rate. Hot peppers contain a chemical called capsaicin; capsaicin gives peppers their spicy taste and helps boost your metabolism as your body works to cool itself down. Spicy meals can boost your metabolism and the boost can last as long as three hours.

Berries and other fruits provide your body with healthy doses of fiber, which works two-fold in helping you to shed fat. First, fiber helps you feel full for a longer period of time, causing you to eat less in the long run. Second, like calcium and complex carbohydrates.

Vegetables are great foods that help you burn fat easily. Some really good ones include asparagus, lettuce and celery. Asparagus helps flush fluids out of your body and contains only 26 calories per cup. Lettuce also minimizes your caloric intake; iceberg lettuce provides only 6 calories per cup. Celery gives only 14 calories per cup. Simply digesting these foods burns more calories than the foods contain, making them very effective fat-burning foods.

It's high time you made your mind up. Cut down on junks, cheese, butter and the likes, eat light at night before eight, exercise regularly, and make a fat burning food roster and keep to it. You will see results with time.

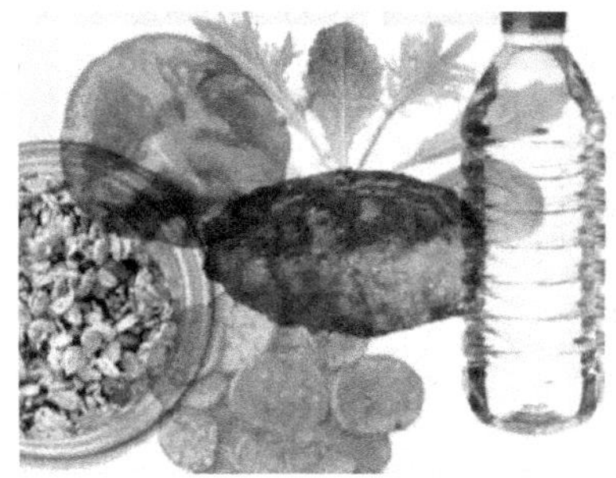

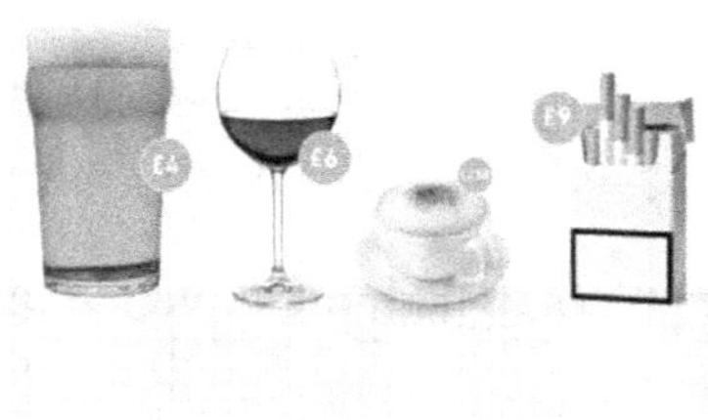

Sometimes, we end up spending money on things that wouldn't improve our health like the picture below depicts.

In the following chapter, we will state the diet plan that will help you lose weight in four weeks. You'd find a week-by-week roster.

CHAPTER TWO

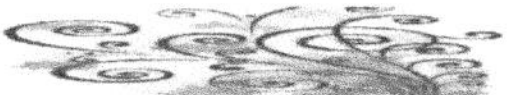

Diet Plan

In this chapter you will find the roster of diets that will speed up metabolism so that you can lose weight in just 28 days.

After 28 days, use the weight scale.

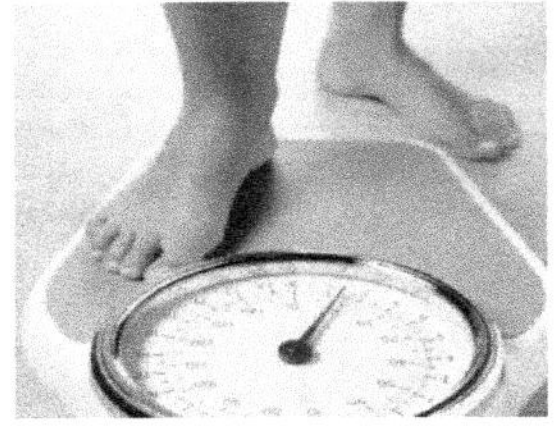

Total Eating Guide

WEEK ONE

Day	Breakfast	Snack	Lunch	Snack	Dinner	Drinks
Monday	Banana Omelette (see recipe)	Handful of nuts and an apple	Protein Salad (see recipe card)	Fruit salad	Stir Fry with turkey (see recipe). Make extra for lunch	Min 2 litres of water / herbal teas
Tuesday	Mango and Cashew Smoothie (see recipe)	Hummus and carrots	Leftovers from last night's dinner	Handful of berries and nuts	Good Old Chili served with cauliflower rice (see recipe). Make extra for lunch	Min 2 litres of water / herbal teas
Wednesday	Protein Pancake (see recipe)	Handful of mixed nuts	Leftovers from last night's dinner	Boiled egg	Chicken Pizza and Sweet Potato Wedges (see recipe) Make extra for lunch	Min 2 litres of water / herbal teas
Thursday	Quinoa with blueberries (see recipe)	Handful of Soy Sauce Seeds (see recipe)	Leftovers from last night's dinner	Snack of choice	Burgers with salad (see recipe). Make extra to freeze	Min 2 litres of water / herbal teas
Friday	Porridge (select choice)	Hummus and carrots	Lunch of choice	Apple and handful of nuts	Chicken Curry (see recipe card)	Min 2 litres of water / herbal teas
Saturday	Sourdough (select choice)	Courgette Pancake (see recipe)	Roast chicken and roasted vegtables	Snack of choice	Dinner of choice	Min 2 litres of water / herbal teas
Sunday	Full English	Carrot and pepper sticks	Protein Salad	Snack of choice	Salmon and Avocado Salsa	Min 2 litres of water / herbal teas

Total Ea **WEEK TWO**

Day	Breakfast	Snack	Lunch	Snack	Dinner	Drinks
Monday	Breakfast shake or any smoothie (see recipe)	Hummus and celery	Protein Salad (see recipe card)	Boiled egg	Lentil Bolognese	Min 2 litres of water / herbal teas
Tuesday	Protein pancake	Handful of nuts	Leftovers from last night's dinner	Snack of choice	Tex Mex Chicken (see recipe)	Min 2 litres of water / herbal teas
Wednesday	Berry Pot (see receipe)	Snack of choice	Leftovers from last night's dinner	Mixed berries	Sweet Potato Cottage Pie (see recipe)	Min 2 litres of water / herbal teas
Thursday	Breakfast Omelette	Handful of berries and nuts	Leftovers from last night	Apple and nut butter of choice	Salmon in Tomato Sauce	Min 2 litres of water / herbal teas
Friday	Chia seed pot (select choice)	Handful of salt and vinegar nuts (see recipe)	Lunch of choice	Cucumber and Hummus	Prawn curry with cauliflower rice	Min 2 litres of water / herbal teas
Saturday	Sourdough (select choice)	Sweet Potato Crisps (see recipe)	Turkey salad (Protein salad) (See recipe)	Boiled Egg	Dinner of Choice	Min 2 litres of water / herbal teas
Sunday	Full English	Fruit salad	Roast chicken and steamed vegetables	Kale Crisps (see recipe)	Chicken Fajitas with parsnip chips	Min 2 litres of water / herbal teas

Total

WEEK THREE

Day	Breakfast	Snack	Lunch	Snack	Dinner	Drinks
Monday	Mango and Cashew Smoothie (see recipe)	Handful of nuts and an apple	Protein Salad (see recipe card)	Fruit salad	Chicken and vegetable bake (see recipe).	Min 2 litres of water / herbal teas
Tuesday	Protein Pancake (see recipe)	Hummus and carrots	Leftovers from last night's dinner	Handful of berries and nuts	Beef Casserole (see recipe). Make extra for lunch	Min 2 litres of water / herbal teas
Wednesday	Banana Omelette (see recipe)	Handful of mixed nuts	Leftovers from last night's dinner	Boiled egg	Butternut Squash Frittata	Min 2 litres of water / herbal teas
Thursday	Berry Pot (see receipe)	Handful of Soy Sauce Seeds (see recipe)	Leftovers from last night's dinner	Snack of choice	Burgers (Veggie Alternative) with salad Make extra to freeze	Min 2 litres of water / herbal teas
Friday	Porridge (select choice)	Hummus and carrots	Lunch of choice	Apple and handful of nuts	Lemon Chicken with courgetti	Min 2 litres of water / herbal teas
Saturday	Full English	Courgette Pancake (see recipe)	Lunch of choice	Snack of choice	Pulled Pork with Sweet Potato Jackets	Min 2 litres of water / herbal teas
Sunday	Sour Dough	Carrot and Pepper Sticks	Roast chicken and roasted vegetables	Handful of Soy Sauce Seeds (see recipe)	Dinner of choice	Min 2 litres of water / herbal teas

Total | **WEEK FOUR**

Day	Breakfast	Snack	Lunch	Snack	Dinner	Drinks
Monday	Breakfast shake or any smoothie (see recipe)	Hummus and celery	Pulled Pork leftovers	Boiled egg	Spag bowl with courgetti (see recipe)	Min 2 litres of water / herbal teas
Tuesday	Banana Omelette	Handful of nuts	Left over spag bowl with salad	Snack of choice	Cajun Chicken and Sweet Potato Wedges	Min 2 litres of water / herbal teas
Wednesday	Porridge (select choice)	Snack of choice	Protein Salad	Mixed berries	Tomato and Egg Bake	Min 2 litres of water / herbal teas
Thursday	Breakfast Omelette	Handful of berries and nuts	Leftover dinner	Apple and nut butter of choice	Burgers and salad (cook extra)	Min 2 litres of water / herbal teas
Friday	Fruit and nut yoghurt	Handful of salt and vinegar nuts (see recipe)	Left over burgers and salad	Cucumber and Hummus	Chicken Curry with cauliflower rice (see recipe)	Min 2 litres of water / herbal teas
Saturday	Salmon and Scrambled Eggs	Sweet Potato Crisps (see recipe)	Lunch of choice	Boiled Egg	Easy roast lamb (see recipe)	Min 2 litres of water / herbal teas
Sunday	2 eggs with mushrooms, bacon and tomatoes	Fruit salad	Left over lamb	Kale Crisps (see recipe)	Salmon and avocado salsa	Min 2 litres of water / herbal teas

In the next chapter, we will discuss extensively on exercises that will speed up body metabolism for weight loss. Then in chapter four you will find the recipes for the above diets.

CHAPTER THREE

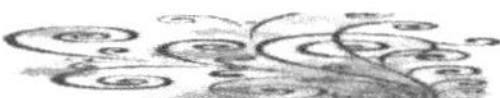

Physical Exercises That Will Hasten Up Body Metabolism

You hate fat and excess weight right? Everyone else does. So learn a few things that will help you trim down completely. Exercises that you will need–

o *Inverted V Pipe Exercise:*

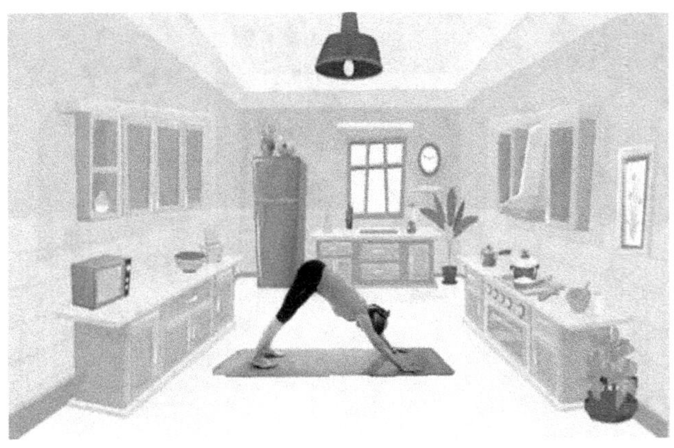

First get a towel as it will help you in the smooth movement of the body. Place your hands on the ground and balance your body on the toes and hands. You will need to pull your legs close to your body, making an inverted V-shape with it. Now, try to push the legs away from your hands by stretching them backward. Pull and push your legs in and out for a few minutes. This movement will work the arms, the core and the lower back.

o *W Leg Lifts Exercise:*

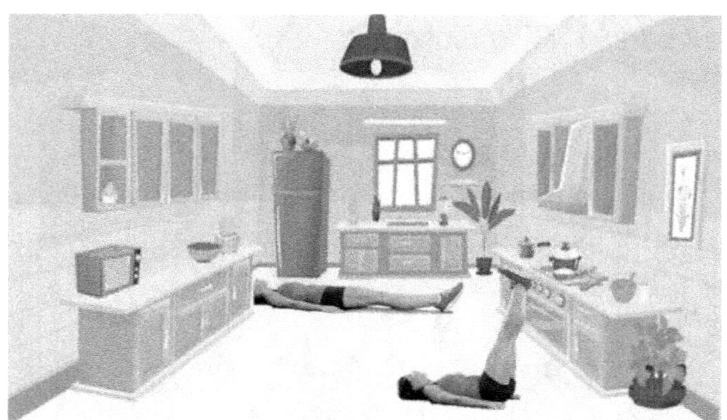

This exercise will work your legs and abs. You will need to lie down on the towel, facing upwards. Put your legs close to each other, and then lift them straight up and bring them to your belly. Put your legs down, but while doing so, stretch them out in the opposite directions and bring them up to your belly. Repeat this same procedure for as long as you can. You will feel a burn in your tummy and legs as you go on. This is undoubtedly the best exercise to lose fat from the lower part of the body.

o *Skipping Exercise:*

This is an easy exercise if you want to lose weight. Both men and women should try it. It is easy to do and entertaining so that you don't get bored. It is the ultimate solution to burning fats in the stomach and thigh. Take a skipping rope and jump for as long as you can. Jumping with both your legs at once will be a much better choice.

You will be warm enough to sweat by the end of this session. Keep your back and knees straight while jumping.

o ***Superman Exercise:***

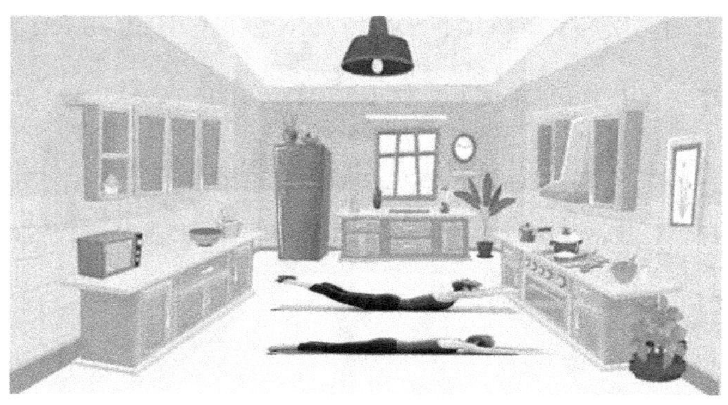

This is a power-packed that works your thighs, abs and lower back. After the W- lifts, turn around and face the ground. Stretch yourself on the ground by keeping your hands and legs straight. You need to lift your chest and thighs off the ground at the same time by balancing yourself on the belly. Keep yourself as straight as possible. Repeat lifting your thighs and chest off the ground for as long as you can. This exercise will give you a flat belly.

o *Single Leg Lift Jump Exercise:*

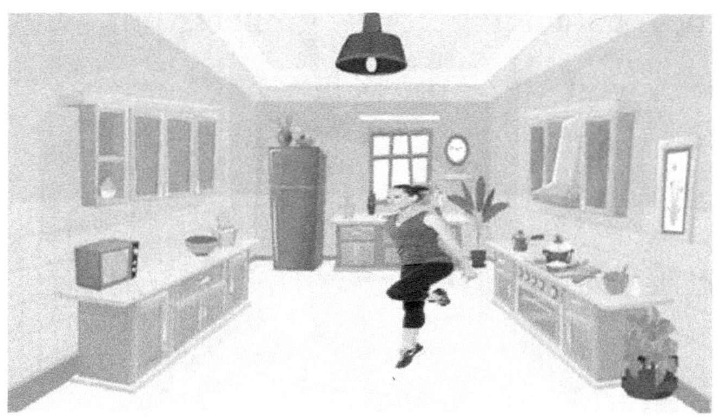

This is one of the most effective workouts to lose weight and tone the body. It works the core muscles and back of the thigh at the same time. It will also help you to gain balance. You need to start by standing straight and lifting the left leg of the ground. Try to touch the ground with your hands and as you come up, you need to jump. Make sure to keep your left leg up all the while. Keep it in a bent position and don't strain it. First you will touch the ground and then jump on your single foot. Do this for 30 seconds. Then shake it off and continue with the next leg. Bend your right knee and continue the same exercise. It may be a little challenging for beginners, but with practice you will pull it off well.

Push up and Knee Kick Exercise (refer to 5 above):

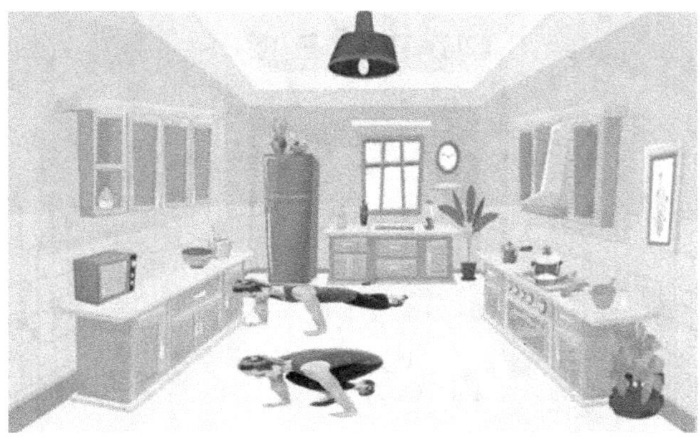

You are conversant already with the traditional push-up but this is a bit advanced and is one of the best home exercises to burn fat. This exercise will work your whole body and will help to lose arm fat. Men are recommended to do a proper push-up. Women can begin with knee push-ups. You need to lie down flat on the ground. Come up to your hands and feet. This is your starting position. You will do just one push up and come back to your starting position. After this you will need to bring your right knee forward to touch your right elbow, and then you will bring your left knee to your left elbow.

CHAPTER FOUR

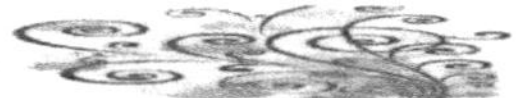

Recipes

This chapter only highlights the recipes of some selected diets. A full recipe for the 4-week weight loss plan is available in the next section of this book. I will begin now to list the recipes starting with Arugula Chicken Salad

ARUGULA CHICKEN SALAD

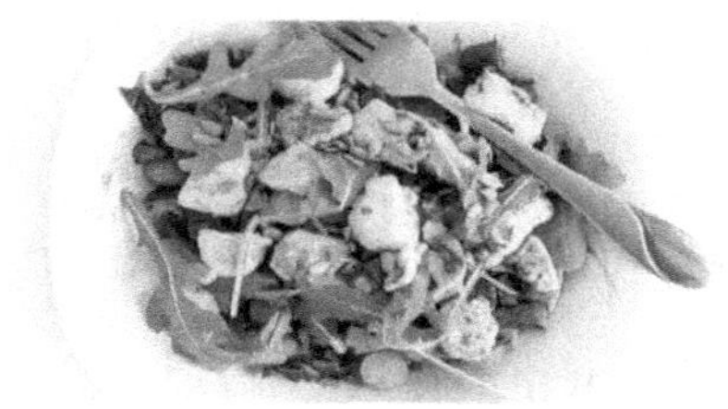

Arugula is a flavorful and notorious vegetable that is low in calories. You will appreciate its long list of health benefits.

What will I need?

- 10 baby carrots, finely chopped

- 1 cup raw arugula

- 8 oz chicken breast, cut into cubes

- 2 tbsp sunflower seeds

- 1 tbsp olive oil

- ½ cup, chopped red cabbage

How will I cook it?

- Put olive oil in a non-stick pan and fry the cubed chicken. Put aside and allow to cool

- Chop baby carrots and red cabbage

- Add cabbage, arugula, and carrots to a large salad bowl

- Top salad with cooled chicken and sunflower seeds

- Add your favourite dressing and enjoy

SOY SAUCE PUMPKIN SEEDS

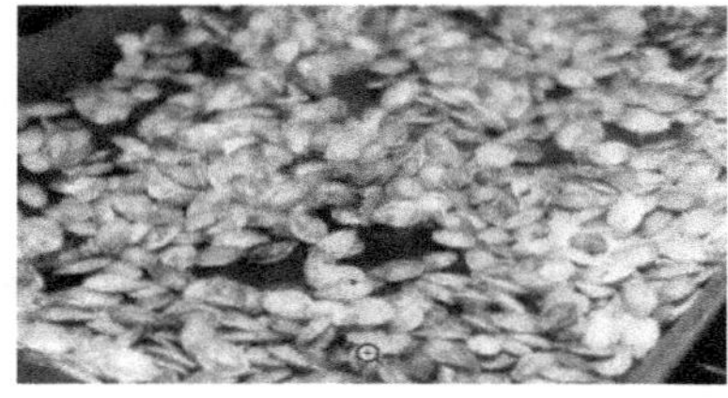

Total time: 35–45 minutes

What will I need?

- 2 tbsp melted butter

- 3 cups pumpkin seeds

- 2 tbsp soy sauce

- 2 tbsp vegetable oil

- Salt (optional)

How will I cook it?

- Preheat oven to 3oo degrees Fahrenheit

- Separate seeds from the pumpkin guts and pour them in a colander. Ensure to rinse very well

- Spread the seeds over a paper towel to dry

- Add vegetable oil, melted butter, and soy sauce and stir together in a bowl

- Spread the seeds on a a baking sheet in a single layer and bake for 35-45 minutes or until crispy and light brown

- Remove from the oven and spread on a paper towel. Pat with additional towels to remove excess oil

- Add salt to your taste and serve.

MANGO AND CASHEW SMOOTHIE

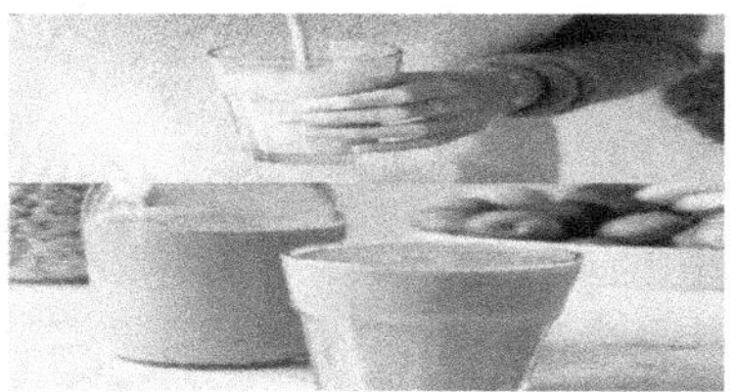

What will I need?

- 1 mango

- 2 ripe bananas

- ½ cups of cashew nuts (80g)

- 2 cups of spinach (60g)

- 2 cups of coconut water or ordinary water, and almond milk (500ml)

- 1 lime

- 1 tablespoon of chia seeds (optional)

How will I cook it?

- Soak the cashews in a glass of water overnight. In the morning drain the cashews and put them in your blender

- Blender the cashew into a smooth cream

- Peel the mango and add just its flesh in the blender with the banana, spinach, cashews, and lime juice

- Blend until it becomes smooth and creamy.

- It is ready to be served

BLUEBERRY QUINOA

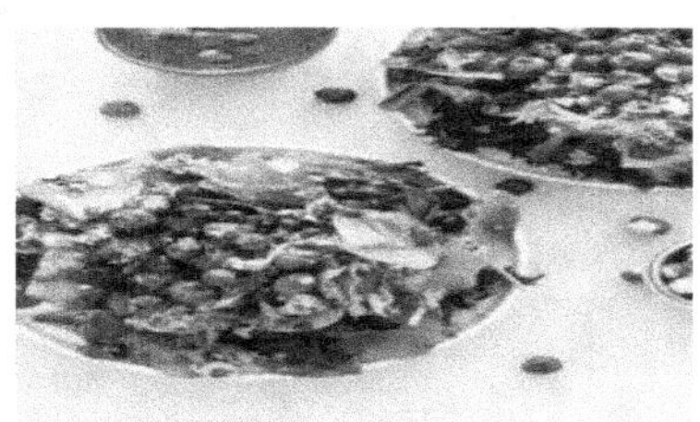

Total time 40 minutes

What will I need?

- 1 cup rinsed quinoa

- 2 cups non-fat milk (or unsweetened almond milk)

- 2 cups Driscoll's Blueberries

- ½ cup chopped pecans

- ¼ teaspoon ground ginger

- 2 tablespoon maple syrup

- ¼ teaspoon ground nutmeg

How will I cook it?

- Place quinoa and milk in a saucepan and boil over high heat, stirring occasionally

- Reduce heat to low and cook for 18–20 minutes or until most of the milk has been absorbed. Ensure it is well covered

- Remove from heat and allow for 5 minutes before you uncover the pan

- Stir in the pecans ginger, nutmeg, blueberries, and maple syrup

- Serve and enjoy

BURGER PATTY SALAD

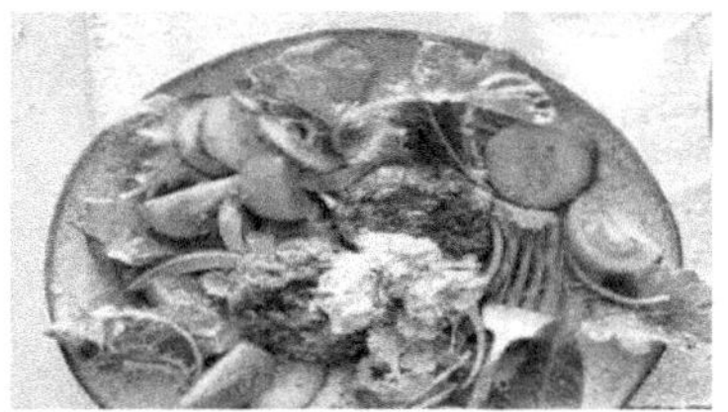

What will I need?

- ¼ cup chopped parsley

- ¾ teaspoon black pepper, divided

- 5/8 teaspoon kosher salt, divided

- ½ medium red onions

- ,¼ teaspoon ground allspice

- 1 large egg

- Cooking spray

- 4 ounces lean ground lamb

- ¼ cup canola mayonnaise

- 2 tablespoon fresh lime juice, divide

- ½ English cucumber

- I tablespoon olive oil

- I medium tomato, cut into 8 wedges

- 1 baby kale leave

- ½ cup plain 2% reduced-fat Greek yoghurt

- 6 ounces 90% lean ground beef

- 2 garlic claves

- ¼ teaspoon ground red pepper

How will I cook it?

- Preheat broiler to high

- Cut the onion half in half and put one of the quarters in a food processor

- Add 2 tablespoons parsley, ½ teaspoon salt, ½ teaspoon black pepper, red pepper, allspice, and garlic. Add lamb, beef and egg. Pulse until all combine well

- Shape beef mixture into 8 patties. Place each patties on a jellyroll pan, coated with cooking spray, and allow to broil for 5-7 minutes or until done

- Mix mayonnaise, yoghurt, 1 tablespoon lime juice, remaining 2 tablespoon parsley, ¼ teaspoon black pepper, and 1/8 teaspoon salt. Grate half of the cucumber into the mixture

- Toss kale with oil and remaining 1 tablespoon juice. Cut remaining cucumber and onion

- Divide kale mixture among 4 plates. Ensure to top each with the cut cucumber, onion, and tomato

- Put 2 patties on each salad and top with yoghurt cream

PORRIDGE

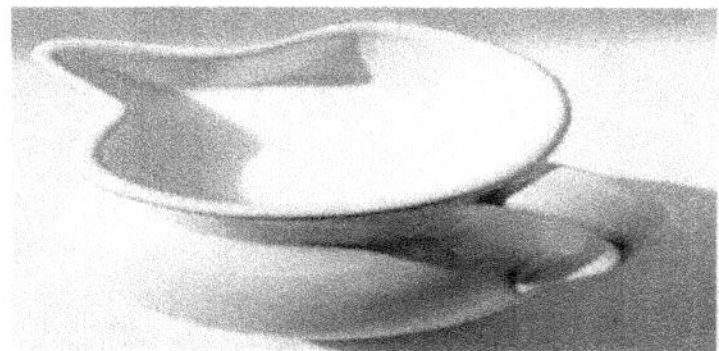

Usually there are several ways to make porridge. This method I'm suggesting to you is the DELIA method

What will I need?

- I teaspoon salt

- Dark brown sugar

- 21/2 oz (60kg) medium oatmeal

- 150ml single cream

How will I cook it?

- Put 570ml water to boil in a medium saucepan then sprinkle in the oatmeal slowly

- Whisk with balloon whisk until the mixture returns to the boil

- Cover the pan and reduce the heat, letting the porridge cook for about 10 minutes

- Add salt, whisk and leave to cook for further 15 minutes

- Bring down the pan and add dark brown sugar over the porridge and let it melt. Pour in the cream.

CHICKEN CURRY

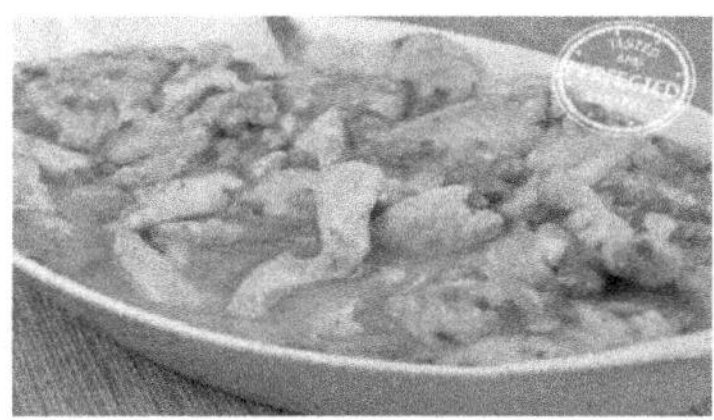

What will I need?

- ¼ cup chopped fresh cilantro\

- ¼ cup plain low fat or Greek yoghurt

- 2 teaspoons sugar

- 1 tablespoon cornstarch

- 2 cups low sodium chicken broth

- 1 tablespoon grated fresh ginger

- 4 minced garlic cloves

- 3 tablespoon vegetable oil, divided

- 1 medium, yellow onion, finely chopped

- Salt and freshly ground black pepper

- 1 pound boneless, skinless chicken breast cut into 4

- 2 teaspoons of curry powder divided into two

How will I cook it?

- Sprinkle ¾ teaspoon salt, ¼ teaspoon pepper, and 1 teaspoon curry powder on the chicken

- Pour 1 tablespoon of oil in a 12-inch skillet over high heat.

- Add the chicken in a single layer and cook until it turns light brown (not well cooked)

- Put the partially cooked chicken in a neat bowl

- Add another teaspoon of oil to the skillet over medium heat. Bring in the onions and stir for about 3 minutes. Then you can stir in the ginger, garlic, and remaining teaspoon of curry powder and cook for about a minute more.

- Whisk the cornstarch and chicken broth together until the cornstarch dissolves. Add thee mix in the skillet together with sugar and 1/8 teaspoon salt. Heat for 5 minutes or until the sauce is thickened

- Add the peas and partially cooked chicken to the skillet, turn down the heat to low and cook till the chicken is done; this can take less than 10 minutes.

- Put off the heat. Stir in the cilantro and yoghurt and season with salt and pepper to taste.

Section 3

TESTED AND TRUSTED: NEWLY FOUND RECIPES

THAT WILL HELP YOU LOSE WEIGHT IN JUST 4 WEEKS

INTRODUCTION

This book is a complete guide and follows up on the book: 'Tested and Trusted: The Little Roster of Diets That Will Shed Excess Weight in 4 Weeks' by Janet Smith. In this book are about twenty different recipes that have been carefully researched and proven to improve quality of life by boosting metabolism for weight loss.

Religiously sticking to a combination of any of the diets will go a long way to help you shed off excess pounds of flesh. The recipes are easy to follow and the ingredients are not out of reach or difficult to get.

The book is easy to read as a result of the non-bulky and straight-to-the-point manner in which recipes are presented. No beating around the bush. No difficult word. No difficult description. This is so because the author realizes how important the recipes are for weight loss and chooses to quickly highlight them. He wants you to reach your goal of losing weight quick.

To benefit maximally from this book, it will be wise to select seven or more different diets that you may wish to incorporate in your food roster.

DIETS AND RECIPES THAT WILL HELP YOU LOSE WEIGHT

I really want to help you shed off excess pounds of flesh. That is why I have taken painstaking efforts in researching and gathering the about twenty recipes that have been proven to boost metabolism and contribute immensely to weight loss.

I am not overweight but I enjoy some of the diets stated therein because of the additional health benefits they are packed with.

Each of the diet is accompanied by pictures to guide you when executing the recipes. Now, let's begin with the recipes.

COURGETTI PANCAKES

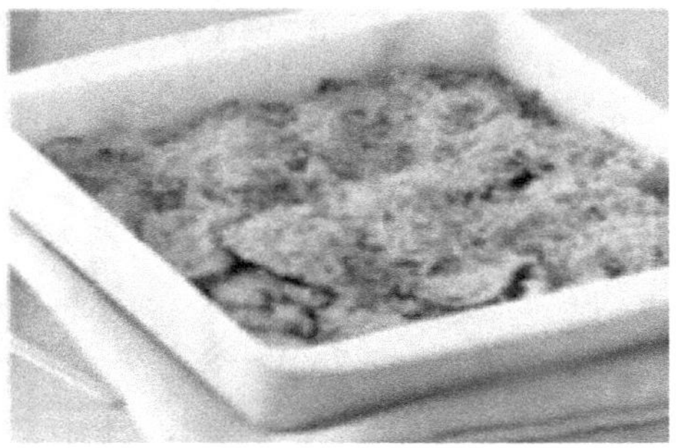

Total time: 10 minutes

What will I need?

- 2 tbsp grated red onions
- 6-8 tsbp plain flour
- 1 teaspoon baking powder
- 1 teaspoon salt h
- ½ teaspoons freshly ground black pepper

- Unsalted butter and vegetable oil
- 2 medium courgettis (375kg)
- 2 extra-large lightly beaten eggs

How will I cook this?

- Preheat oven to 150 degrees
- Grate the courgettis into a bowl. Stir in the eggs and onions immediately
- Stir in 6 tbsp of flour, salt and pepper, baking powder
- Heat a large sauté pan over medium heat and melt ½ tbsp oil and ½ tbsp butter in the pan
- When the butter becomes hot, lower the heat to medium-low and add soup spoons of batter into the pan. Allow the pancakes to cook for 5 minutes or until each side turns brown

- Put the pancakes on a sheet pan and keep warm in the oven. Ensure to wipe out the pan with a paper towel.

- Add some more butter and oil into the pan to continue to fry until you have used the rest of the batter.

The pancakes are ready. Serve them hot.

SOURDOUGH BREAD

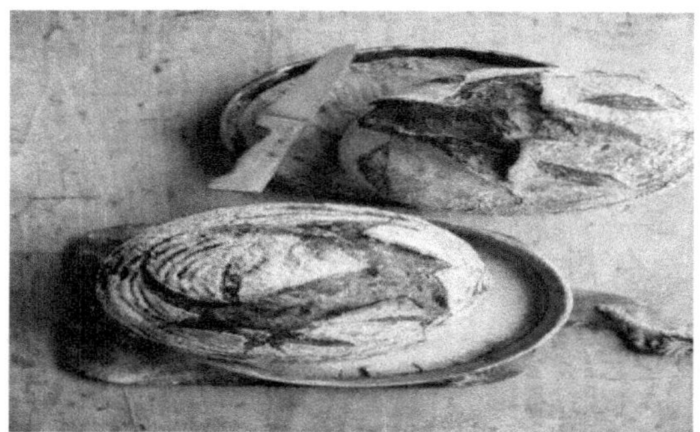

Total time: it is relative

What will I need?

- 100g sourdough leaven (made with starter)
- 300g water
- 100g of stoneground organic whole meal flour

- Semolina for dusting the bottom of the baking surface

- 400g organic strong white flour

- 10g fine sea salt mixed with about 15g of cold water

- 250g rice flour mixed with about 25g stone ground white flour to be used in dusting your banneton

How will I bake it?

- Whisk your water and starter in a large bowl and mix well. Add all the flour and mix together until the ingredients form a large ball

- Cover with a damp cloth and let the dough rest on the side for between 45 minutes and 2 hours

- Add the salt mixed with water and dimple your fingers in the dough so that the salty water will distribute evenly in the dough. Allow for 10 minutes

- Lift and fold your dough over, doing a quarter turn of your bowl. Do it three times every thirty minutes

- Shape the dough into a ball and place into a round banneton dusted with flour. Dust the top with flour cover with a damp tea towel

- Allow your dough until is 50% bigger. Then transfer it to the fridge and allow to prove for 8–11 hours

The following morning

- The next morning, preheat your oven to 220 degrees for 35 minutes before baking. Place your baking stone in the oven and a large pan underneath (or try to use a Dutch oven).

- Once the oven has reached full h you are using a Dutch oven. Allow to bake for an extra 20 minutes or until you see a desired color eat, carefully take out the baking stone and dust with some semolina flour so that the bread does not stick. Put the dough on the baking stone and slash with blade; this determines where the bread will tear as it rises. Allow to bake for 1 hour.

- Reduce the heat to 180 degrees and remove the lid if. I usually prefer dark brown; it tastes better

KALE CRISP WITH PERMESAN CHEESE

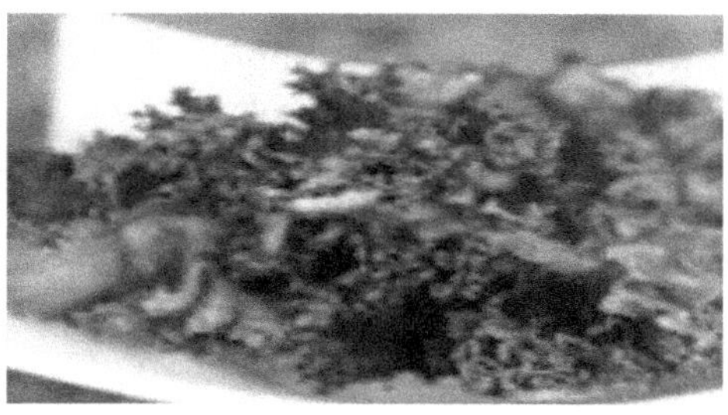

Total time: 20 minutes

What will I need?

- 1 bunch kale
- 1 teaspoon seasoned salt
- 1 teaspoon olive oil
- Parmesan cheese
- Lime juice

How will I cook it?

- Preheat your oven to 180 degrees/ Gas 4 Line a baking tray with a baking parchment
- Carefully remove with a knife, the leaves from the thick stem and tear into bite size pieces
- Wash and dry kale with a salad spinner, then sprinkle the kale with olive oil and salt
- Allow to bake for 10-15 minutes until the edges turn brown
- Remove the kale from the oven into a bowl and drizzle with lime juice. Place the parmesan cheese on top and serve

TEX MEX CHICKEN

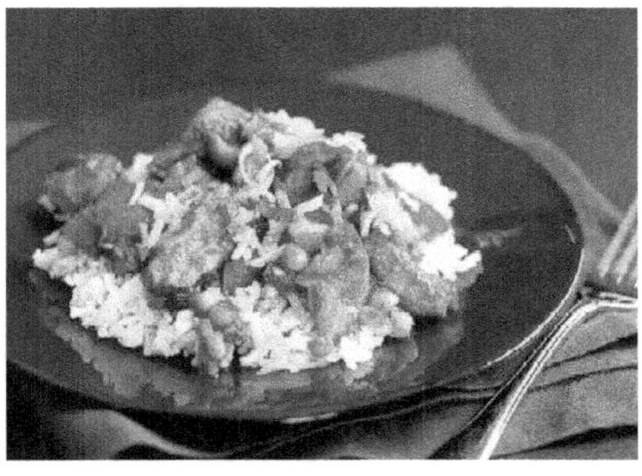

Total time: 5 hours

What will I need?

- 2 tbsp Taco seasoning mix
- Boneless skinless chicken breast, cut into 1-inch- wide strips
- Chunky salsa
- 2 tbsp flour

- 1 green and 1 red pepper, cut into 1-inch-wide strips
- 1 cup frozen corn
- 2 cups hot cooked long-grain white rice
- 2 green onions, sliced

How will I cook it?

- Toss chicken with seasoning mix and flour in a slow cooker sprayed with cooking spray. Add peppers, salsa and corn, and mix lightly. Cover with lid
- Cook on low heat for 6–8 hours or on high heat for 3–4 hours
- Stir chicken mixture
- When it is ready, serve over rice with onions and cheese

PARSNIP CINANAMON CRISPS

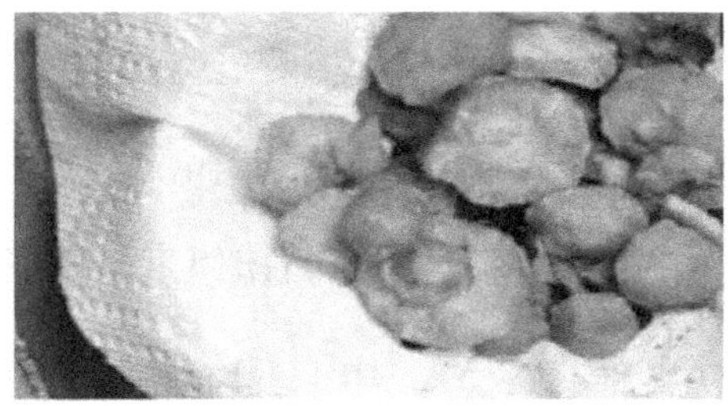

Cook time: 20 minutes

What will I need?

- ¼ cup vegetable oil
- 1 large parsnip, peeled and sliced very thin
- I teaspoon of cinnamon
- ½ of kosher salt

How will I cook?

- Preheat oven to 475 degrees

- Peel and slice the parsnip to be really thin

- Pour the vegetable oil, cinnamon and salt in a large zipper plastic bag. Seal the bag and use your hand to mix so that the oil and spices can combine

- Add the parsnips, and press until the spiced oil coats all the parsnips evenly

- Lay the parsnips flat on a large cookie sheet that is covered with asilpat.

- Cook for 10 minutes, flip, and cook for another 7 minutes until it is crinkly and the edges turn light brown

Serve immediately

CLASSIC BEEF CASSEROLE

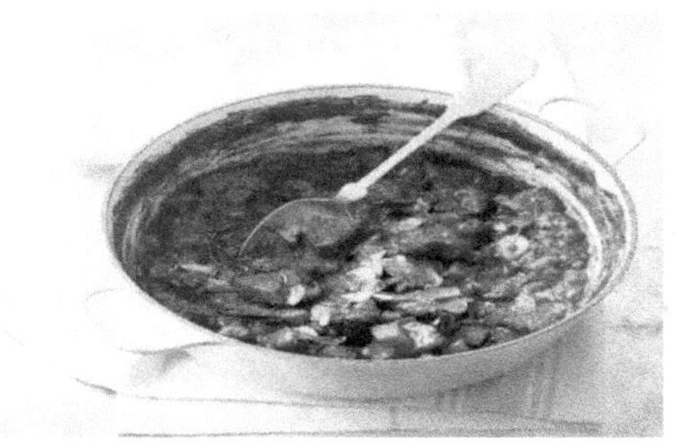

Total time: 35 minutes

What will I need?

- 3 garlic cloves, finely chopped
- 2 tbsp. tomato purée
- 2 celery sticks, finely chopped
- 2 onions, finely chopped
- 1kg braising steak, sliced into 4cm cubes

- 2 large carrots, sliced into 2cm cubes

- 2 tbsp plain flour

- 1 tbsp vegetable oil

- Unsalted butter, 40g

- 2 tbsp chopped oregano or parsley leaves

- 250ml red win

- 500ml beef stock

- 400g chopped tomatoes

How will I cook it?

- Measure out half the oil and half the butter in a large casserole, and place over medium heat. When hot, fry the beef in 3 batches until they turn brown. Put the browned or fried beef in a bowl with a slotted spoon.

- In the remaining oil in the casserole melt the rest of the butter over a low heat. Add the celery, onions, garlic, and carrots. Stir for 5 minutes until the onions have become soft.

- Add the flour and tomato purée, and keep stirring for 1 minute.
- Put the beef and its remaining juices in the casserole together with the wine and allow over high heat to cook for 2 minutes or until they become thickened.
- Reduce the high heat to medium. Add the stock and chopped tomatoes. Season and stir well. Cover and allow simmering for one and half hours. You can occasionally stir in the last 30 minutes.
- When the sauce becomes thick and the beef tender, stir in the herbs and adjust the seasoning.

Your beef casserole is ready to be served.

Tips: you can vary the flavorings by using a rich, tasty ale such as Guiness or stout instead of the red wine. The chocolate stout is preferable with beef.

SWEET POTATO CRISPS

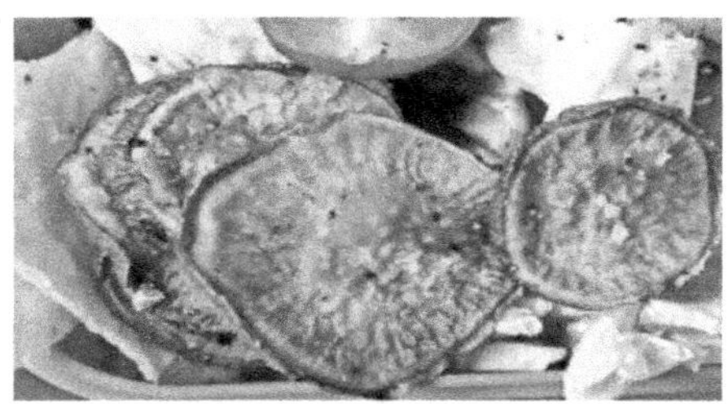

This is a great lunchbox filler and vegan too. I make this every once a week. Sometimes I prefer to eat sweet potato crisps 2 hours before bedtime. I enjoy it with a cup of pear juice.

Total time: 20 minutes

What will I need?

- Fresh potato
- I tbsp oil

How will I cook it?

- Put oven to a heat of 200c. add butter in a skillet and allow to hot

- Thinly slice the sweet potato and toss into the hot oil

- Fry for 10-15 minutes until they become crisp.

SPAGHETTI BOLOGNESE WITH COURGETTI

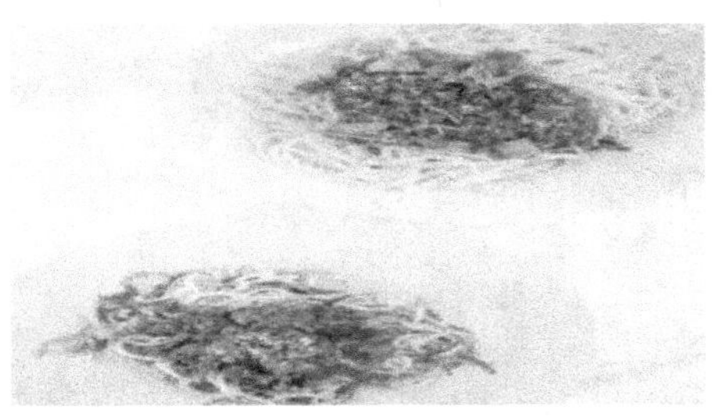

Total time: 20 minutes

What will I need?

- 3 cloves garlic, finely chopped

- 2 onions, finely chopped

- 500g beef mince

- 500g pork mince

- 3 tbsp tomato purée

- 2 small carrots, finely chopped

- 1 tbsp balsamic vinegar

- 2 cans chopped tomatoes

- 1 bay of leaf
- 1 tbsp dried basil
- 1 tbp dried oregano
- 1 teaspoon sugar
- 1 teaspoon marmite
- 2 sticks celery, finely chopped
- Handful sliced mushrooms
- Spash of red wine
- 500ml beef stock
- Olive oil
- Salt and pepper\

How will I cook it?

- Mince the pork and beef together in a pan and fry, stirring continuously for 5-10 minutes to ensure it doesn't clump up into big chunks of mince.
- When they turn brown, empty the meat on a plate and drain off excess oil

- Add a little olive oil in the pan and fry the carrots, onions, celery and mushrooms until softened. Add the garlic and fry for an extra 1 minute.

- Put the meat back into the mix and fry, stirring continuously until everything thing mixes together

- Add the balsamic vinegar, tomato purée, sugar, and marmite and fry for another 1 minute so that the alcohol can evaporate.

- Add the 2 cans of chopped tomatoes, bay leaf, and beef stock. Season with a little salt and pepper and allow simmering over low heat for 50 minutes or until the sauce becoming thick and nice. Ensure to check it every once in a while so that it doesn't stick.

How to make Courgetti

I recommend 1 large courgetti for you alone because it does shrink down as you cook it.

- Heat butter in a pan or skillet and add in the courgettis. Add a little salt and fry until it is soft to your liking (I enjoy mine quite soft).
- Drain it off in a basket. Your courgetti is ready.
- Serve with the spaghetti Bolognese and grate over some freshly ground black pepper and fresh basil.

BERRY POTS

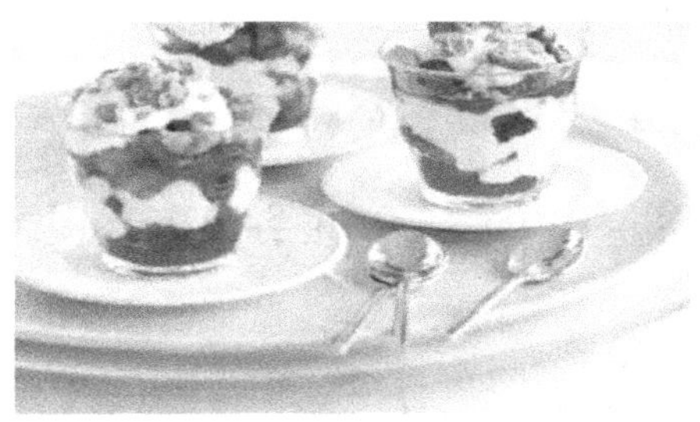

Total time: 10 minutes

What will I need?

- 4 tbsp double cream, lightly whipped or Greek yoghurt
- 8 amaretti biscuits
- 150ml fresh custard
- 300g mixed berries
- Juice 2 clementines or satsumas
- 2 tbsp strawberry jam

How will I cook it?

- In a bowl, mix the jam and citrus juice together. Stir in the berries cut half the berries between 4 gasses and top with the custard, the remaining berries and the cream

- Crumble over the biscuits and serve.

CHILI AND CAULIFLOWER RICE

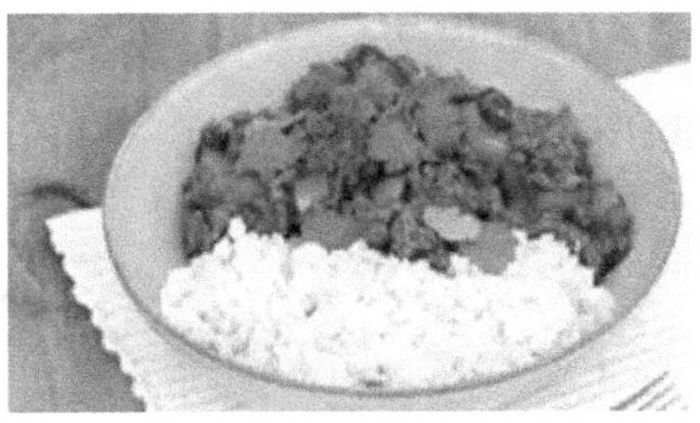

Total time: 60 minutes

What will I need?

- 3 garlic cloves, peeled and finely chopped

- 1 onion, peeled and finely chopped

- 1 teaspoon ground cinnamon

- 2 teaspoon ground cumin

- 4oog can chopped tomatoes

- Coriander springs (optional)

- 2 cauliflowers, broken into florets

- 2 red peppers with seeds removed, cut into small pieces

- Salt and ground black pepper

- 400g can red kidney beans in chili sauce

- 500g lean beef mince (5% fat or less)

- 1 teaspoon cayenne pepper or paprika

- Chunky salad like cucumber, tomato, and red onion, to serve

How will I cook it?

- Place a large, non-stick pan over medium heat and add the onion and garlic. Stir-fry for 2 minutes or so before adding the cayenne pepper, cinnamon, cumin, paprika, and beef mince. Stir-fry for about 6 minutes

- Add the peppers and tomatoes. Ensure to season well and cook over low heat for about 25 minutes

- Put in the beans and stir to mix well. Allow to cook for another 10 minutes
- Place the florets in a food processor in batches. If you do not have a food processor, you may consider grating the cauliflower
- Put the finely chopped cauliflower in a microwaveable dish, well covered, and cook for some 3 minutes. With a fork fluff the cauliflower up and serve.
- Put down the chili from the heat and serve with the rice and garnish with the salad.

Tips: The chili can be frozen without the rice

PROTEIN PANCAKES

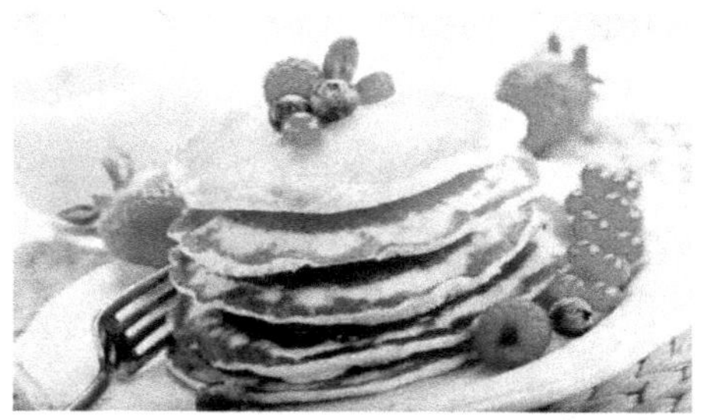

Total time: 12 minutes

What will I need?

- 1 large egg
- 50g porridge oats
- ¼ teaspoon baking powder
- Light cooking spray
- 100ml milk
- 25g whey protein powder

How will I cook it?

- Add the oats to a blender and crush until it is like flour. Add the protein powder, baking powder, cinnamon, milk, and egg to the blender and grind all together until you have a texture like pancake batter

- Put a little oil in a frying pan and place over medium heat

- Pour in the mixture in the pan, using ¼ of the total mixture for each protein pancake

- Shake the pan in a circular motion so that the batter coats the surface evenly

- Allow the pancake fry for a maximum of 1 minute or until the bottom becomes light brown. Then flip over and cook the other side. Repeat this process for the remaining protein pancakes.

BANANA OMELETTE

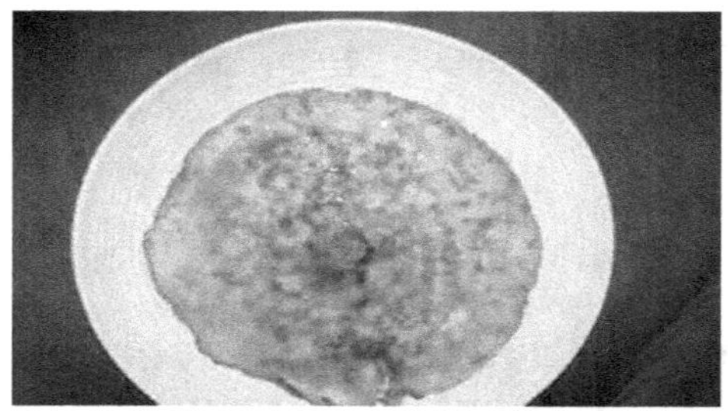

Time Taken: 5 minutes

What will I need?

- 1 banana
- 2 teaspoon of plain flour
- 3 tablespoon of honey
- 2 teaspoon of butter
- 1 egg
- ¼ cup milk

How will I cook it?

- Stir flour, milk and egg until mixture is smooth

- Marsh the banana and add to the mixture. Ensure to mix until it blends with the mixture

- Add butter in a frying pan and place over medium heat. When the butter melts, put in the mixture all at once.

- Cook both sides until light brown

- Serve with honey on top

ARUGULA CHICKEN SALAD

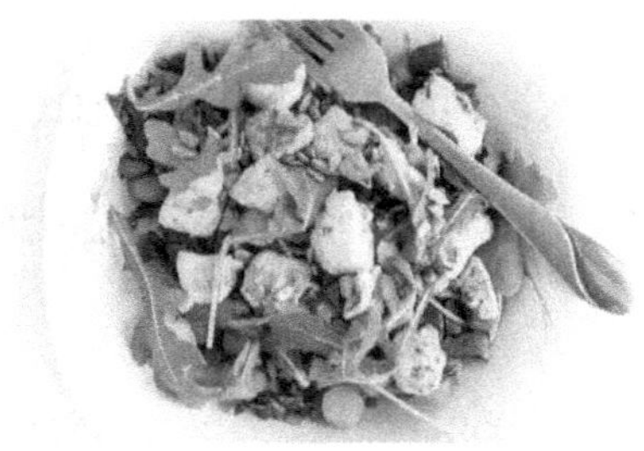

Arugula is a flavorful and notorious vegetable that is low in calories. You will appreciate its long list of health benefits.

Total time: 35 minutes

What will I need?

- 10 baby carrots, finely chopped
- 1 cup raw arugula
- 8 oz chicken breast, cut into cubes
- 2 tbsp sunflower seeds

- 1 tbsp olive oil
- ½ cup, chopped red cabbage

How will I cook it?

- Put olive oil in a non-stick pan and fry the cubed chicken. Put aside and allow to cool
- Chop baby carrots and red cabbage
- Add cabbage, arugula, and carrots to a large salad bowl
- Top salad with cooled chicken and sunflower seeds
- Add your favourite dressing and enjoy

SOY SAUCE PUMPKIN SEEDS

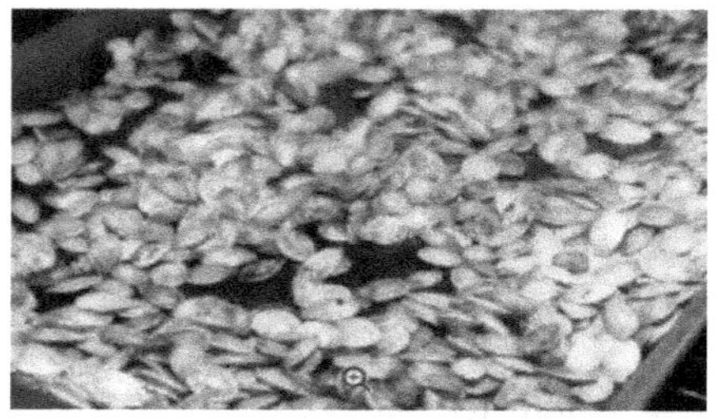

Total time: 35–45 minutes

What will I need?

- 2 tbsp melted butter

- 3 cups pumpkin seeds

- 2 tbsp soy sauce

- 2 tbsp vegetable oil

- Salt (optional)

How will I cook it?

- Preheat oven to 3oo degrees Fahrenheit
- Separate seeds from the pumpkin guts and pour them in a colander. Ensure to rinse very well
- Spread the seeds over a paper towel to dry
- Add vegetable oil, melted butter, and soy sauce and stir together in a bowl
- Spread the seeds on a a baking sheet in a single layer and bake for 35-45 minutes or until crispy and light brown
- Remove from the oven and spread on a paper towel. Pat with additional towels to remove excess oil
- Add salt to your taste and serve.

MANGO AND CASHEW SMOOTHIE

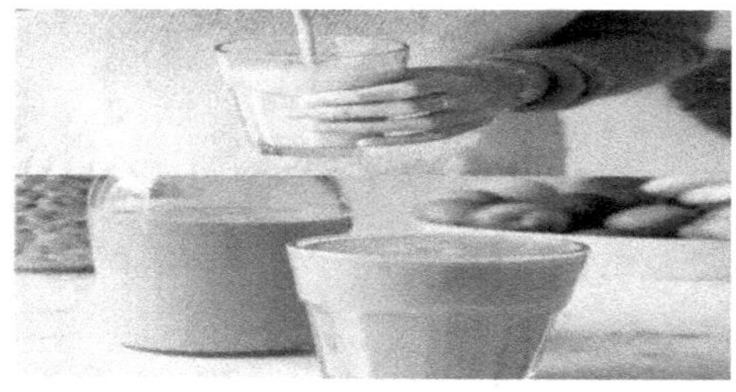

Total time: 10 minutes

What will I need?

- 1 mango
- 2 ripe bananas
- ½ cups of cashew nuts (80g)
- 2 cups of spinach (60g)
- 2 cups of coconut water or ordinary water, and almond milk (500ml)
- 1 lime
- 1 tablespoon of chia seeds (optional)

How will I cook it?

- Soak the cashews in a glass of water overnight. In the morning drain the cashews and put them in your blender
- Blender the cashew into a smooth cream
- Peel the mango and add just its flesh in the blender with the banana, spinach, cashews, and lime juice
- Blend until it becomes smooth and creamy.
- It is ready to be served

BLUEBERRY QUINOA

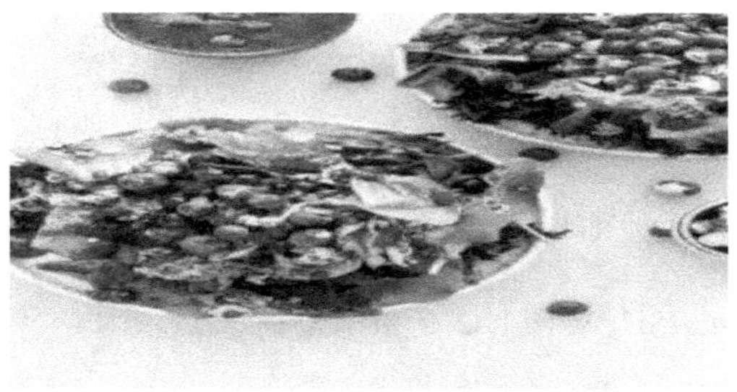

Total time: 40 minutes

What will I need?

- 1 cup rinsed quinoa
- 2 cups non-fat milk (or unsweetened almond milk)
- 2 cups Driscoll's Blueberries
- ½ cup chopped pecans
- ¼ teaspoon ground ginger
- 2 tablespoon maple syrup
- ¼ teaspoon ground nutmeg

How will I cook it?

- Place quinoa and milk in a saucepan and boil over high heat, stirring occasionally
- Reduce heat to low and cook for 18–20 minutes or until most of the milk has been absorbed. Ensure it is well covered
- Remove from heat and allow for 5 minutes before you uncover the pan
- Stir in the pecans ginger, nutmeg, blueberries, and maple syrup
- Serve and enjoy

BURGER PATTY SALAD

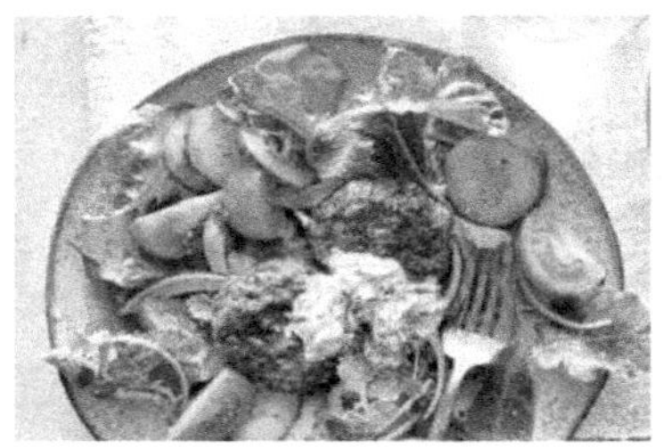

Total time: 30 minutes

What will I need?

- ¼ cup chopped parsley
- ¾ teaspoon black pepper, divided
- 5/8 teaspoon kosher salt, divided
- ½ medium red onions
- ,¼ teaspoon ground allspice
- 1 large egg
- Cooking spray
- 4 ounces lean ground lamb

- ¼ cup canola mayonnaise

- 2 tablespoon fresh lime juice, divide

- ½ English cucumber

- I tablespoon olive oil

- I medium tomato, cut into 8 wedges

- 1 baby kale leave

- ½ cup plain 2% reduced-fat Greek yoghurt

- 6 ounces 90% lean ground beef

- 2 garlic claves

- ¼ teaspoon ground red pepper

How will I cook it?

- Preheat broiler to high

- Cut the onion half in half and put one of the quarters in a food processor

- Add 2 tablespoons parsley, ½ teaspoon salt, ½ teaspoon black pepper, red pepper, allspice, and garlic. Add lamb, beef and egg. Pulse until all combine well

- Shape beef mixture into 8 patties. Place each patties on a jellyroll pan, coated with cooking spray, and allow to broil for 5-7 minutes or until done

- Mix mayonnaise, yoghurt, 1 tablespoon lime juice, remaining 2 tablespoon parsley, ¼ teaspoon black pepper, and 1/8 teaspoon salt. Grate half of the cucumber into the mixture

- Toss kale with oil and remaining 1 tablespoon juice. Cut remaining cucumber and onion

- Divide kale mixture among 4 plates. Ensure to top each with the cut cucumber, onion, and tomato

- Put 2 patties on each salad and top with yoghurt cream

PORRIDGE

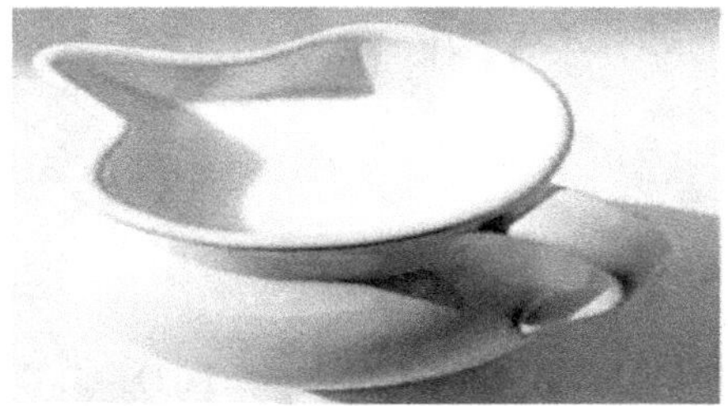

Usually there are several ways to make porridge. This method I'm suggesting to you is the DELIA method

Total time: 30 minutes

What will I need?

- I teaspoon salt
- Dark brown sugar
- 21/2 oz (60kg) medium oatmeal
- 150ml single cream

How will I cook it?

- Put 570ml water to boil in a medium saucepan then sprinkle in the oatmeal slowly

- Whisk with balloon whisk until the mixture returns to the boil

- Cover the pan and reduce the heat, letting the porridge cook for about 10 minutes

- Add salt, whisk and leave to cook for further 15 minutes

- Bring down the pan and add dark brown sugar over the porridge and let it melt. Pour in the cream.

CHICKEN CURRY

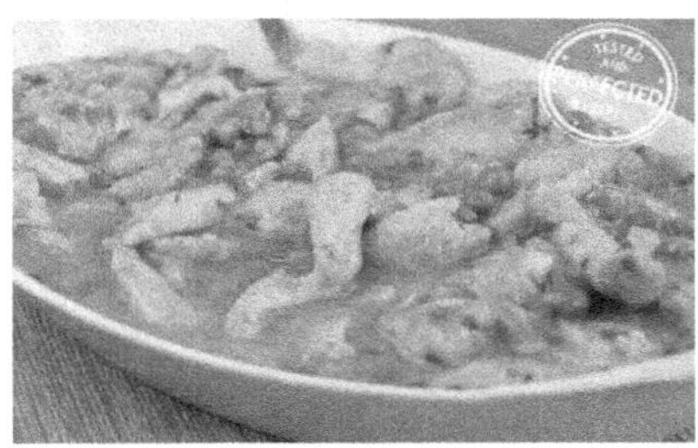

Time taken: 15 minutes

What will I need?

- ¼ cup chopped fresh cilantro\
- ¼ cup plain low fat or Greek yoghurt
- 2 teaspoons sugar
- 1 tablespoon cornstarch
- 2 cups low sodium chicken broth
- 1 tablespoon grated fresh ginger
- 4 minced garlic cloves
- 3 tablespoon vegetable oil, divided

- 1 medium, yellow onion, finely chopped

- Salt and freshly ground black pepper

- 1 pound boneless, skinless chicken breast cut into 4

- 2 teaspoons of curry powder divided into two

How will I cook it?

- Sprinkle ¾ teaspoon salt, ¼ teaspoon pepper, and 1 teaspoon curry powder on the chicken

- Pour 1 tablespoon of oil in a 12-inch skillet over high heat.

- Add the chicken in a single layer and cook until it turns light brown (not well cooked)

- Put the partially cooked chicken in a neat bowl

- Add another teaspoon of oil to the skillet over medium heat. Bring in the onions and stir for about 3 minutes. Then you can stir in the ginger, garlic, and remaining teaspoon of curry powder and cook for about a minute more.

- Whisk the cornstarch and chicken broth together until the cornstarch dissolves. Add thee mix in the skillet together with sugar and 1/8 teaspoon salt. Heat for 5 minutes or until the sauce is thickened

- Add the peas and partially cooked chicken to the skillet, turn down the heat to low and cook till the chicken is done; this can take less than 10 minutes.

- Put off the heat. Stir in the cilantro and yoghurt and season with salt and pepper to taste.

Section 4

REBRAND YOUR LIFE: DRINKS THAT WILL BOOST METABOLISM IN 28 DAYS

INTRODUCTION

I work nine hours every day, six times a week, but I'm up and doing because the word 'ill health' has not really been part of my dictionary. I don't expect ill health, anyway. Why should I, especially with my strong routine of Garlic bread and tea in the mornings, and peer juice with enough milk, for dessert. You see, I just discovered whole 'bundle' of nutrition facts about some foods and drinks, and I believe you'd need scme at your fingertips.

The drinks and their health benefits are clearly stated. For those who are really interested in weight loss, this short read is essential. You will appreciate the simplicity of the recipe.

It is a fact that what goes inside reflects on the outside. This book, seeks to assist people improve their health, by virtue of what they drink. The drinks discussed can go a long way in improving your health and managing overweight. More so, the recipes are easy to follow. Why not begin now, to drink something that will help you live long?

As you follow the instructions in this book, you will trim off excess pounds of flesh, and be better able to cope with stress and any element that might hamper your quality life. Good health to you.

CHAPTER ONE

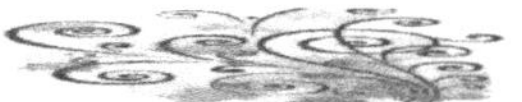

PEAR JUICE

Simply speaking, any drink made with pear as the major ingredient is pear juice. Some may decide to add milk and a bit of honey to improve on the look. While there those who really like it when mango and pineapple is crushed with it in the electric juicer. However, before I go on to tell you the 'how to', take some time to look at the health benefits packed inside pear juice,

Benefits of taking pear juice

Pear juice is not a commonly known drink. But it is quite tasty. If you give it a try, you will always want it again. Some of the benefits of drinking pear juice include;

- Low caloric content:

The common complaint that people have about other fruit juice is the high caloric content in them which is obtained from natural sugars. But pears are among the foods with the lowest calorie. An average pear juice contains about 58 calories (just one glass). The nutrition provided by pears is quite immeasurable and it gives you a feeling of satisfaction. So people who desire to lose weight can add pears to their diet. It is both a high-energy and high- nutrient food with little impact on weight gain.

- Maintaining the skin:

If you want to prevent premature aging, pear juice is right for you. Pear fruit has high a high amount of Vitamin C, copper and Vitamin K. These nutrients give the fruit juice the ability to fight harmful radicals and thus protect the skin cells from damage. There is toning of the skin and the formation of lines near the eyes and lip area is prevented or stopped.

- Prevention of cancer:

One health benefit of pear juice is that it can prevent the development of cancer. The fibers from pear juice can bind themselves with bile acids and a special group of bile acids known as secondary bile acids. The high amounts of secondary bile acids present in our intestines can increase the risk of colorectal cancer. But the fiber in pear helps to reduce the concentration in the intestine, and lower the risk of developing cancer. Taking pear juice also reduces the risk of stomach cancer. The various key components in fiber phytonutrients and cinnamic acids have cancer fighting properties. A study done in Mexico City showed that 2 fruit servings of pear can decrease the risk of gastric cancer. Esophageal cancer is a dangerous type of cancer but pear juice can reduce the risk and effect. A large scale study was done by the National Institute of Health and American Association of Retired persons, which showed that pear was a key food that reduced the risk of esophageal cancer.

- Antioxidant activity:

Pears contain a good amount of antioxidants just like other fruits. These antioxidants are helpful in fighting various diseases and illnesses in the body. Antioxidants help eliminate the free radicals which gather in the body through a process called cellular metabolism. These free radicals can change healthy DNA into cancerous cells which can have a devastating effect. So the antioxidant components of Vitamin A, Vitamin C, and beta-carotene which are found in pear juice can help the body get rid of dangerous diseases

- Digestive and intestinal health:

Pear juice has an important role in digestion. One glass of pear juice provides about 18% of the daily body requirement of fiber which are a strong agent for digestive health and function. The majority fiber in pear is non-soluble polysaccharide. This means it acts as a bulking agent in the intestines. It gathers the food and adds bulk to it so that the food can easily pass through the intestines. It also stimulates the secretion of gastric and digestive juices so that the food can move smoother in a digested state. More so, bowel movement is put under control thus reducing the chances of constipation.

The pear juice also binds itself to the cancer-causing and free radicals in the colon and helps to protect the organ from harmful effects. It is noteworthy that Pear juice has about 6.5% fructose and 1.3% sucrose. Free fructose isn't absorbed properly. It becomes fermented in the large intestines thus resulting in the production of SCFA (Short chained fatty acid) which leads to the absorption of a small energy in the colon. This explains why we use pear juices in the treatment of constipation.

- Birth defects:

Folate is another valuable nutritional components found in pear juice. Research has shown that folic acid correlates positively with the reduction of neural tube defects in newborns. So, pregnant women are encouraged to drink pear juice.

- Potassium content:

Pear juice is a good source of potassium. Potassium is a good vasodilator (it opens the blood vessels). It helps to lower the blood pressure and the strain on cardiovascular system and thus stops the formation of clots. It also increases the blood flow to all parts of the body. Low blood pressure leads to lower chances of different cardiovascular diseases like strokes, atherosclerosis, and heart attacks. Potassium also helps to regulate the fluids in the body and keeps different organs hydrated.

- Bone health:

Pear juices contain minerals in high amount. These minerals include phosphorous, manganese, magnesium, copper and calcium. This means that the effects of bone loss and serious bone conditions like osteoporosis and general weakness of the body are reduced.

- Skin, eyes and hair:

Vitamin A is one of the most important vitamins in the body. Pears have high amount of vitamin A and other components like leutin and zea-xanthin. They function as a good antioxidant and reduce the effects of aging on skin. Pear juice also reduces hair loss, cataracts and other health conditions that come with aging.

- For weaning children:

Pear juice is so helpful for weaning children (stopping the supply of breast milk and introducing a young child to an adult's diet). The reason is that it is hypoallergenic. So it doesn't result in any digestion problems. The fruit juice can be served cold to children. But it shouldn't be given to children with diarrhea.

How to make Pear juice:

Pear juice can be made with an electric juicer. The juicer makes it easy for you to experiment with different flavors for pears. Here is how to make some delicious pear juice at home:

1. You should select firm and bright pears, with skin that is free of bruises and imperfections. Firm pears produce better juice. You will end up making a puree when the pears are too soft.

2. Ensure to wash the pears in cold water. Wash the surface area to remove any kind of dirt.

3. At this point you will need to cut the pear and remove any seeds and stem attached to it. Cut the pear into little chunks before you put into the electric juicer. (Chop any other ingredients you want to put with pear juice.). You can add fruits like pineapple, mango, apple and vegetables like celery, spinach, broccoli and carrots.

4. Put additional ingredients into the juicer and run the juicer. I usually enjoy adding a lot of condensed milk to enhance the taste.

At this point, you can remove the juice compartment and serve the pear juice. Enjoy the pear juice fresh.

How Best To Store:

The best way to store pear juice is to put it in a refrigerator. You may wish to use an air tight container, freezer bag, Mason jar, or ice cube tray.

When the pear juice is taken out of storage, it might be a bit thicker. You may dilute it with a lighter drink or water. You can also defrost the juice and make pear jellies.

CHAPTER TWO

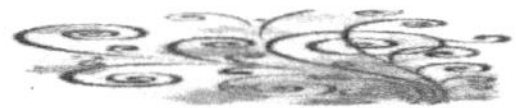

COFFEE

Let me ask you; do you really know coffee? I'm sure you are probably nodding or smiling by now. But then what do you know about coffee? Do you know that around the world, countless numbers of people prefer to start the day with a warm cup of coffee? I take coffee in the morning too. But when I was studying for a bachelor's, I would drink a cup of coffee at night to keep me alert during night studies. Drinking coffee is a great way to get together with family and friends! Can you imagine the joy of sipping up during such friendly atmosphere? It lifts our moods and relieves stress. More so, coffee has an enticing aroma and distinctive flavor (you know what I mean).

But did you know that besides the enticing aroma, reviving taste and distinctive flavor, a cup of coffee contains a solid bunch of health benefits? Let me start by telling you ten reasons why coffee is splendid and absolutely good for you.

Reasons You Should Start Taking Coffee

First of all, Coffee does not interfere with calcium absorption. There is a common misconception that taking coffee can lead to calcium loss from the body. But current study has shown that coffee has no negative effect on bone health. And of course, strong and healthy bones are a result of diets rich in calcium. Why not prepare your coffee with a full glass of milk? This will certainly help you meet your calcium needs.

Second of all, soluble Coffee is 100% coffee. Soluble coffee is processed using pure coffee beans and water without additives. It's the selection of beans and the distinctive roasting process that provides its special aroma.

Third of all, Coffee helps you learn better and stay more alert at work. Studies have proved that people who take coffee are relaxed and more interested in their work. The caffeine content in coffee helps to restore and maintain alertness, thereby improving performance and enhancing your mood. It is the perfect brew if you want to be alert and active at work. When studying, coffee helps improve attention and wakefulness, increasing attentiveness and by that it facilitates learning. (While I was studying for a bachelor's degree, I made a second class upper because Nescafe kept me alert at night; the time I studied best).

Fourth of all, Coffee is the number one source of antioxidants. Current research has shown that coffee contributes significantly to your daily total antioxidant intake. Antioxidants help protect your cells from oxidation and your body from cancer, heart disease, and premature aging!

Fifth of all, Coffee enhances your physical performance. According to research, caffeine plays a role in contributing to better physical performance. This could help athletes perform better at endurance exercises of short and long durations, as well as strenuous routines

Sixth of all, Coffee can help protect your skin. Your skin is constantly exposed to harmful external factors such as UV ray, which can affect the health of your cells and cause them to damage. But with the antioxidant-rich properties of coffee, your skin can fight the damaging effects of the sun and prevent wrinkles as well.

Last of all, Coffee can help ease headaches. Research suggests that a cup of coffee may help to relieve you of migraine symptoms and even stop it if consumed at the very initial stage of the headache. This is because substances like caffeine constrict blood vessels and help counter the throbbing effects of blood vessel dilation in your head.

Whether you choose a caffeinated or decaffeinated blend, you will still get all the benefits of antioxidants since both have similar content. You can drink 3-4 cups a day. For those who take coffee, the recommendation for moderate consumption is 300 mg of caffeine daily or the equivalent of 3-4 cups of soluble coffee. 1 cup of soluble coffee has less than 2 calories. In fact it is what you add to the coffee that adds calories. So remember to have your cup with less sugar and low fat milk.

CHAPTER THREE

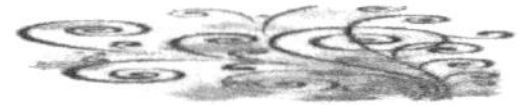

GREEN COFFEE

Green coffee is currently among the world's most popular weight loss supplements. As the name implies, this supplement is extracted from the same beans people use for brewing coffee. The only difference is that green coffee beans are raw, unroasted coffee beans. The roasting process seems to destroy some of the healthy, natural chemicals in the beans. Because of media attention, green coffee has become a popular supplement for weight loss.

Benefit of taking Green coffee:

9. Green coffee also seems to help lower high blood pressure in some people. One small study in people with mild high blood pressure showed benefit over the placebo

10. Some research shows green coffee may help with weight loss. A few small studies found that people taking green coffee lost 3 to 5 pounds more than people who weren't. Green coffee may act by lowering blood sugar and blocking fat buildup.

Quantity of Green coffee to take:

The active ingredients in supplements vary widely from maker to maker. This makes it hard to set a standard dose. Ask your doctor for advice. Before you venture into green coffee, please tell your doctor about any supplements you're taking, even if they're natural. That will help your doctor check on any potential side effects or interactions with medications.

Wait a minute. Have you heard about Coffee beans? Like any other beans they are complex in nature. There are some 40 different substances responsible for the taste and health properties of coffee. However, the main thing I want to tell you relates to Green coffee beans. It is no longer uncommon to hear about Green coffee beans and the health benefit. Green coffee beans are the coffee beans in their natural form. The truth is that these beans are the same coffee beans that you consume daily in the form of drink. The only difference is that Green coffee beans are unroasted. When these beans are later roasted for commercial use, they turn brown and lose Chromogenic Acid which is largely responsible for weight loss. So if you are looking forward to the weight loss benefit of coffee you should use the green coffee beans in the unroasted form.

The taste of green coffee beans is very much different from the roasted beans that you usually make. The flavor you will get from the green beans is not very strong and hence you will get little watery taste. Those having problems with the taste of green coffee can take green coffee extract because of its improved taste.

It is possible to find the roasted coffee beans around you but to get the fresh green coffee beans; you may need to go online where you will find the best.

Before you make green coffee drink from unroasted coffee beans, keep the following in mind:

- Ensure to use the best quality Arabica coffee beans to get the best taste. You can also use the one grown by organic farming.
- If you are allergic to coffee or have any tolerance issues, please check with your doctor before consuming this drink.

Ingredients For Making Green Coffee:

- Green Coffee Beans (Arabica or similar) 20 g
- Hot water 300 ml or 2 cups
- Honey or sugar (this is optional)

There are two methods for making green coffee drink. Whatever method you want to opt for, just endure that the coffee beans are unroasted.

Method 1-

How to prepare coffee using green coffee bean powder:

4. Grind the green coffee beans in a grinder to get the fine powder depending on your liking and the available appliance. Green coffee beans are unroasted beans, so they are really hard to grind. You will require heavy duty grinder.

5. Divide the powder into two cups and add in hot water. Water should be hot but not boiling (about 90°C).

6. Leave for 10 minutes and then drain with fine sieve to get your drink ready to sip.

7. You may add sugar or honey if you like but for those looking for the health benefits; it is recommended to drink it plain.

Method 2–

How to prepare green coffee using whole green coffee beans:

Preparing coffee from whole beans is usually a time consuming method. You may prepare this coffee in large batches. Soak the beans overnight in water.

- Heat the mixture of soaked beans and water. When it is boiled, simmer the mixture on low flame for 15 minutes. Stir occasionally.

- Ensure the mixture is cool before sieving it to remove beans from the mixture.

- The concoction you are now having is concentrated. So you may add filtered or distilled water to dilute the concoction.

- If you have prepared this in a large batch then you can store the rest in a deep freezer to be used within 3 days.

- Add cardamom or any other additives. This will add more taste to this healthy drink.

Whether you use the first or second method, make sure you take one cup after each meal for best results.

As you take Green Coffee for weight loss, you should keep the following facts in mind.

The caffeine in green coffee, just like the caffeine in brewed coffee, can cause stomach upset, headache and anxiety. However, the major health risks associated with drinking green coffee includes:

1. Glaucoma

2. Diabetes

3. High blood pressure

4. Irritable bowel syndrome

4. Osteoporosis

5. Bleeding disorders

Talk to your doctor if you have any medical conditions before using a green coffee supplement. There is no reliable evidence about its safety of green coffee, so it is not recommended for children or for pregnant or nursing mothers.

Green coffee interacts with many medicines. Some of these include stimulants, blood thinners, and medicines for:

1. Menopause

2. Depression

3. Schizophrenia

4. Heart problems

5. Weak bones

6. Lung diseases

ADVICE: Do not take green coffee along with herbal stimulants or other supplements with caffeine.

Section 5

POACHED EGGS: THESE LITTLE SECRETS MEAN A LOT

Introduction

Poached eggs are quite awesome. In this little book, you will learn a whole lot about poached eggs; the method of preparation, the hidden health benefits, why poaching eggs is better than any other methods of cooking eggs. In the last chapter, you will be motivated to start a restaurant, selling poached eggs and garlic bread or pasta.

Whether you can poach eggs or not this book will be of immense benefit to you. It is a short, simple, timely, and interesting read.

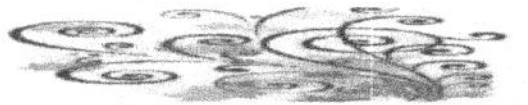

Chapter one

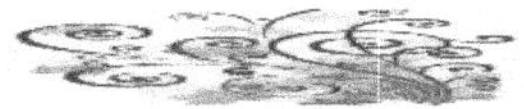

EGGS AND THE METHODS OF POACHING

In my small town where poultry business is very common, we eat eggs every day. We buy one and half crate every two week, consuming them in egg sauce, egg roll, egg this egg and egg that. I still remember how my mother, a couple of years ago, used to say a day should not go by without an egg in your stomach. It was her philosophy, a strong one for that matter. And when only three or four eggs were left, she'd bound into my room. You have to go to the grocery store. We have no eggs. I always went to the grocery store to buy them.

It is true that we are advised to eat eggs every day. Some eat eggs every once in two days, some three, some four. It is based on choice for some and pocket for some. At least, the good thing is that a week did not pass without eggs on the table. However, how often do you consume poached eggs? Do you really know that poached eggs are far better than frying, baking, or scrambling eggs? In case this may surprise you, not to worry, this book has come to your aid with solid facts about the various methods of cooking eggs.

Let me start by giving you a run down about eggs. But before then, I recommend the following books to you because I believe you care about your health and you might want to try something healthy.

Facts on eggs

- Eggs are known to contain cholesterol
- Eggs are one of the most consumed animal products in the world

- Eggs are one of the best sources of proteins

Health Benefits of Consuming Eggs

I will quickly list some of the health benefits of eggs as a reminder

> - Egg keeps you feeling full much longer than cereals. The protein and fat in egg can sustain your energy level.
> - Eating eggs for breakfast can help in weight loss.
> - Eggs help to lower the risk of heart diseases.
> - Eggs help strengthen eyesight especially because of its lutein content.

> They nourish the shin. Little wonder there are a lot of body creams out there with eggs as the major constituent. .

> The Vitamin D content helps to keep the bones and teeth healthy.

> Eggs have biotin which is essential for energy, metabolism, and strengthening the immune system.

> Eggs contain folic acid which is essential for blood formation especially during pregnancy.

> Selenium is another national value of egg. This helps in protecting cells from oxidative damage.

Methods of cooking eggs

Eggs can be cooked in several ways the most of which involves; frying, baking, scrambling, and poaching. We will discuss each under sub headings..

1. Frying eggs

This method of egg preparation involves using heated butter. You can heat the butter in a nonstick skillet. In this method, the egg is heated in oil until it flattens and turns light brown.

What you will need

Eggs

A skillet or frying pan

Butter

Pepper

Onions

The preparation process usually involves the following:

5. Crack the number of eggs you desire to use, pour into a bowl and begin to stir.

6. Heat butter in a skillet or frying pan for 1 minute.

7. In the eggs you can slice in onions and peppers or whatever you prefer, and keep stirring.

8. When the butter is sufficiently hot, pour in the mx.

9. Wait for 2-3 minutes, turning the edges every once in a while until it turns light brown.

10. The process is quite simple right? Of course, but how healthy is fried eggs to you? Well, you'd need to hold on a bit lets highlight the other methods.

2. Baking

In this method, an oven is required. It is also referred to as shirring. It is quite tasty an easy is the first method. This method of cooking eggs involves the temperature of about 163 degrees.

What you will need

- Eggs
- Salt and pepper
- Milk
- Tbsp

The preparation process involves the following:

- Heat oven to about 325 degree Fahrenheit
- Break and slip the quantity of eggs you desire into a custard cup
- Add milk to your taste
- Sprinkle pepper and salt to your taste
- Leave in the oven for about ten minute.

- When the whites are set and the yolks begin to thicken, not very hard, bring it down. Your baked egg is ready to be served.

3. Scrambling

Scrambled eggs are a bit more tasking than the aforementioned methods.

What you will need

- Eggs
- Butter
- Milk
- Salt and pepper
- Skillet or frying pan

The following are the processes involved in scrambling eggs:

- Beat two eggs together, add two tablespoon of milk, water, pepper and salt if you want.
- Blend together.

- Heat a small amount of butter in a 5-inch omelet pan or skillet over medium heat.

- When it becomes hot, pour in the egg mixture. As the eggs begin to set, pull them across with a turner.

- Keep cooking, pulling, lifting, and folding eggs until they are thickened. Endeavor not to stir randomly.

4. Boiling

This is the simplest method of cooking eggs. In this method, eggs are boiled with their shells. Unlike the other methods, all you need to do is slip in as much eggs as you want into pot of water. Let it cook for 2-3 minutes before taking it down.

My own mother was used to this method. When she did not boil them the alternative was frying. So I grew up thinking that frying and baking were the only methods of cooking eggs. But this came to change later on. Now the method I carefully researched on is the next.

5. Poaching

This is a unique way of preparing eggs. It involves boiling eggs without their shells

What you will need

Eggs

Milk

Wine

Tomato juice

Onion (no compulsory)

Skillet

How to prepare poached eggs

- Heat about 4 inches of water, milk, broth, tomato juice, onions, and wine. You may use any other liquid aside wine, in a deep skillet.

- Make sure you adjust the heat to keep the liquid summering.

- Break eggs into a container cne after the other, do not stir.

- Your container must be close to the hot liquid.

- Slip the eggs into the liquid. Allow to cook until the yolks thicken and the whites are completely set. This process should not go beyond 3 to 5 minutes.

- Afterward, lift the out the eggs ith a slotted spoon, drain the eggs. Some people may add salt or vinegar to the liquid because they want to enhance coagulation. But that is not necessary.

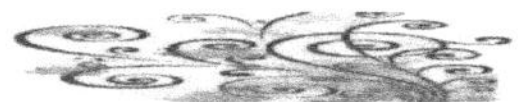

Chapter Two

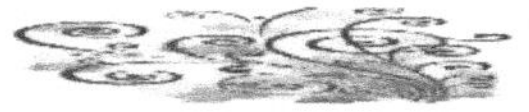

POACHED EGGS AND YOUR HEALTH

I scramble eggs every once in a while. Sometimes I fry too. But I poach eggs most of the times. My mother does not know much about poaching eggs. The conventional way of frying or boiling them in their shells was what I grew up with. You may be wondering why I chose to write about poached eggs when I didn't grow up with it. Well, I learnt something new along the line.. Let me quickly tell you why.

Why poaching eggs is healthier than the other methods

1. Unlike the egg boiled with its shell, poached eggs have a significantly low level of calories. Besides you have lots of additional nutrients as a result of the other things added to poached eggs.

2. Compared to fried and baked eggs, poached eggs contain higher calories. The calories in poached eggs are not too high or too low. You system can benefit from the balance.

3. A poached egg can supply nearly six grams of high quality protein, over 4.5 grams of unsaturated fat band a high amount of Vitamin D, anti-oxidant compounds and man more nutrients which are really important the brain to function properly.

4. Poached eggs are cooked in boiling water of at about 212 degrees Fahrenheit. But baked

or fried eggs go beyond that. The heat involved in frying or baking eggs can easily reach 400 degrees. High temperature cooking is unhealthy as it produces toxic compounds known as AGEs. Some of these toxins oxidize body tissue. By poaching eggs you help prevent the fats in the yolk from being oxidized. The moment you expose an egg's yolk to air, its cholesterol becomes oxidized. Though only a small percentage of oxidized cholesterol is retained in the body, it is best to avoid this oxidized cholesterol as consumption can lead to heart diseases.

The basic principle that you cannot underestimate in cooking eggs is to use a medium to low temperature. Do not over heat and do not over low. Either way, you'd be making the egg yolk shrink and rubbery. Some may assume that cooking eggs in extreme temperature will kill bacteria. Sure, it will but you'd be endangering your health. So when boiling eggs watch until the whites are firm and the yolk thickened before you take them down. The required temperature is 70 degrees.

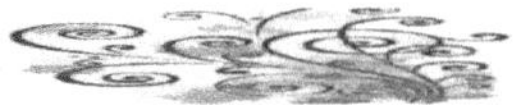

Chapter Three

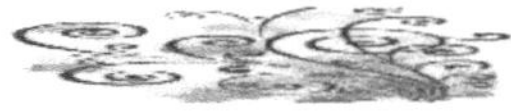

TOOLS FOR POACHING EGGS

The major kitchen equipment you'd need for poaching eggs are

- Egg Slicer
- Egg Cooker

8. Egg Slicer

This is a good egg preparation utensil. It is used to perfectly slice peeled hard boiled eggs into several even units. It is quite fast. If you like the look of equal shapes in your plate of salad, then you should get an egg slicer. There are some really good brands of egg slicers like the ChefsGrade Slicer, Tablesto Slicer, Westmark Slicer, New Star

Slicer, and so on. Except you have one in mind already, theses brands are awesome..

9. Egg cooker

The value of these cookers can never be underestimated. There cookers however, for boiling, scrambling, or poaching eggs. The eggs are ready quickly, without stress. Bedsides, you save yourself the trouble of calculating time as a result of the built-in timers. Some cookers have alarms to signify when you bring down your eggs. Others shut down automatically when the eggs are well cooked.

So then before you decided to buy any egg cooker, or change the one you already have, decide on what you will use it for; scrambling, boiling, or poaching. Next, decide on how big or small you want the cooker to be. If you are cooking for you and your small family, you may need a cooker that can hold four to six eggs. Most cookers can hold up to twelve eggs. You may consider this if you own a restaurant.

Caring for Your Egg preparing Equipment

- Clean after use
- Do not leave cookers on electricity when not in use
- Switch off cooker when the eggs are ready

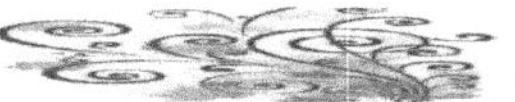

Chapter Four

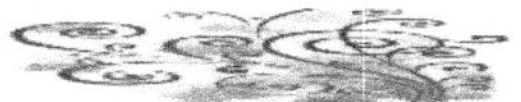

GARLIC BREAD WITH POACHED EGG

Have you eaten bread before? You're probably smiling because the question has a rhetoric answer. But what about garlic bread, have you eaten it? Now you're probably thinking!

Owing to the surplus benefit garlic offers, eating garlic bread reduces the risk of becoming overweight and providing your body with sufficient amount of carbohydrates. Instead of butter, you can use olive oil margarine. Ensure to use fresh garlic since, it is the healthiest in that condition. Eating garlic bread is not so common in many countries of the world. But if you have eaten it, you are missing a whole lot of delicious snack. It can be eaten with tea, millet pap, bean cake, coffee, or as you may please. I enjoy eating garlic bread with groundnut. That is enough lunch to hold me until dinner time. Once, we tried it with coconut and it tasted nice too. The good thing is that you feel a kind of spicy taste that could send you to seventh heaven. I know by now, you are having some saliva stuck in your mouth. Please swallow it while I tell you how eating garlic bread can be a plus to your health.

Health benefits of garlic bread

Since the major ingredient in garlic bread is garlic, highlighting the benefits of garlic invariably explains why garlic bread is helpful.

- Garlic improves your immune system. So eating garlic bread could be what you need to fight against cold.

- There is adequate content of Vitamin B1, B2, B6, B12 in garlic so it implies invariably that eating enough garlic bread with sum to give your body the needed B- complex.

- There is presence of copper, phosphorus, manganese, potassium, and calcium in garlic bread making it your favorite ingredient for bread.

- Garlic has anti-inflammatory properties which is absolutely good for you.

- Garlic bread can protect your heart.

- Garlic has anti-fungal properties so you can be sure that eating garlic bread can prevent fungus overgrowth.

- Research has proven that garlic consumption can help prevent or reduce chances of lung cancer. Does eating garlic bread now sound nice to you?

- Garlic also reduces your chances of brain cancer.

Ingredients for making Garlic Bread:

- 1 16-ounce loaf of Italian bread or French bread
- 1/2 cup (1 stick) unsalted butter, softened
- 2 large cloves of garlic, smashed and minced
- 1 heaping tablespoon of freshly chopped parsley
- 1/4 cup freshly grated Parmesan cheese (optional)

How to make Gaelic Bread:

1. Heat oven to 350°F.
2. Cut the bread in half, horizontally. Mix the butter, garlic, and parsley together in a

small bowl. Spread butter mixture over the two bread halves. Place on a sturdy baking pan (one that can handle high temperatures, not a cookie sheet) and heat in the oven for 10 minutes.

3. Remove pan from oven. Sprinkle Parmesan cheese over bread if you want. Return to oven on the highest rack. Broil on high heat for 2-3 minutes until the edges of the bread begin to toast and the cheese (if you are using cheese) bubbles. Watch very carefully while broiling. The bread can easily go from un-toasted to burn.

Remove from oven, let cool a minute. Remove from pan and make 1-inch thick slices. Serve immediately with the poached eggs (Use the same process above in making poached eggs).

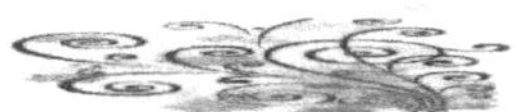

Chapter Five

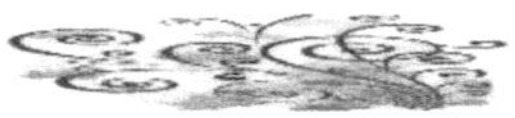

THE NUTRITIOUS PASTA WITH POACHED EGGS

It is high time you learned this short way of preparing nutritious Pasta. Many people fail to eat healthy deserts. For example Macaroni (pasta) is not prepared to nourish the body with what it needs. That is why I took my time to share with you how to prepare healthy pasta

What you need:

- 8 ounces whole-wheat angel hair pasta

- 2 tablespoons of extra-virgin olive oil, or vegetable oil
- 4 or 5 pieces of garlic
- 3 plates of shredded, peeled sweet potato
- 1 large red bell pepper, thinly sliced
- 1 plate of diced plum tomatoes
- 1/2 cup water
- 2 tablespoons of chopped fresh parsley
- 1 tablespoon of chopped fresh tarragon
- 1 tablespoon white-wine vinegar, or lemon juice
- 1/2 tablespoon of Salt or as desired
- 1/2 plate crumbled goat cheese.

How to prepare:

- Boil a large pot of water
- Cook pasta until it is a bit tender (4 to 5 minutes or according to package directions).

- Meanwhile, place 1 tablespoon of oil and garlic in a large skillet.

- Cook over medium heat, and stir occasionally, until the garlic is sizzling, 2 to 5 minutes.

- Add sweet potato, pepper, tomatoes and water and cook, stirring occasionally, until the pepper is tender-crisp, 5 to 7 minutes. Remove from the heat; cover and keep warm.

- Drain the pasta, reserving 1/2 cup of the cooking water.

- Return the pasta to the pot. Add the vegetable mixture, the remaining 1 tablespoon oil, parsley, tarragon, vinegar (or emon juice), salt and cheese; toss to combine.

- Add the reserved pasta water, 2 tablespoons at a time, to achieve the desired consistency. Allow to cook for about 2 minutes.

Your nutritious pasta is ready to be served with the poached eggs.

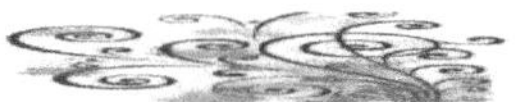

Chapter Six

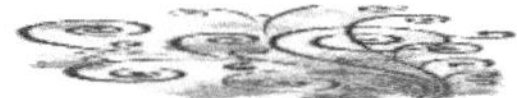

POACHED EGGS AND BACON SALAD

Bacon Salad is also known as Salad Lyonnaise. It is a traditional French salad typically from Lyon. It is prepared with hot bacon, curly endive, and freshly poached eggs.

Ingredients required

- 2 tablespoons of strips bacon
- 2 poached eggs
- 2 teaspoon butter
- 2 slices of Italian or French bread

- Two handful of fresh frisee lettuce

- 2 Tbsp olive oil

- 2 Tbsp wine vinegar

- 1 teaspoon of chopped shallots

- 1 teaspoon of Dijon mustard salt

- Lastly, you'd need some peppers.

How to Prepare

- The first thing you need to do is too cook the four strips of bacon over a medium heat. For about five minutes.

- Take it down from the heat and let the fat rain out. Once it becomes cool enough, chop.

- Slice the French or Italian bread into cubes. Then toast them over medium heat with two teaspoons of melted butter. Do not stir, except that you can turn the sides every once in a while.

- The next thing to do is to poach the eggs.

- Lastly, put the chopped cooked bacon, shallots, and frees lettuce on a salad plate. In a separate bowl mix the vinegar, salt, pepper, olive oil together.

Spread the dressing over your salad and place the poached eggs on top.

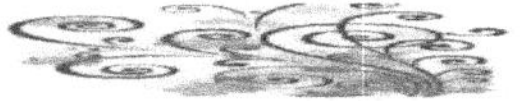

Chapter Seven

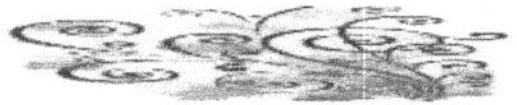

MAKING MONEY WITH POACHED EGGS

I decided to try out what I learnt about poached eggs at home, one day. You see, it is one thing to read and learn. It is absolutely another to put to practice what has been learned. And of what use is knowledge to you if you don't make practical use of it?

The day I made poached eggs, my mother came nagging that I was trying to waste eggs. She was rather unlettered and ordinary in nature so I understood her worries.

"Do not worry mom," I calmly said to her and she briskly walked out of the kitchen.

When the poached eggs were ready, I served them on our dining table and beckoned on my mother. It was just the two of us in the house. So you can imagine how lonely the house was.

My mother sat on one chair while I sat opposite her.

"Mom, taste it, you will like it," I said.

My mother stretched out her hand into the ceramic and jabbed some with a fork. She bobbed her head and smiled.

"I never knew I was missing a whole lot," she said.

The following day, I bought flour from the grocery shop and made Garlic bread which was an awesome compliment for poached eggs. My mother kept eating with pleasure.

"People will like this," she said. "It's like a new food, a good new food."

She was right. With all the perfect benefits of garlic and egg and thr other ingredients, the doctor was only faraway. The combination was perfect.

Eventually we decided to create a business out of this. We opened a small restaurant in our small town were we started making scrambled and poached eggs with garlic bread and pasta for people.

It is from this business that we got the money to renovate our house which was already old, with cracks advertising itself on the wall.

You can make Money by being creative with food

You see, there is nothing really bad with you playing around with food. Test different ideas. The only thing is, it has to be a healthy mix. One day, you will stumble on something really crazy. If there is something you can cook with a unique style, why not think of getting into the big picture of selling it to people. There are thousands of people out there who are looking for new foods. I can assure you, they will be willing to pay for something new. Not just new, it should be nutritious. Like the experience of Kentucky, the founder of Kentucky Fried Chicken, you could break into success.

My final word to you on this is read business motivational books. It can be a boost. Eat well. Stay healthy.

Legal Disclaimer

This book and the content provided therein are simply for educational purposes and to serve as a guide to those who plan to or are already on a ketogenic diet. Though the advice of the author has proved to be effective for some people, it does not offer a general solution to complications relating to ketogenic diet and weight loss. It is not to be seen as a medical book.

The information provided therein is solely for educational purposes and is not intended to treat any serious medical condition. The content of this book should not be used in place of advice from your physician. In other words, before you begin this diet plan, check with your doctor.

The transmission and receipt of information therein does not construe a therapist–patient relationship between you and the writer. However, you can freely contact the author for questions regarding the recipes discussed.

ABOUT THE AUTHOR

Janet Smith lives with her mother in a small town. They run a restaurant for a living. When she is not at the restaurant, she writes extensively on topics pertaining to food and nutrition.